A Colour Atlas of
The Surgery and Management of Intestinal Stomas

L. R. Celestin, F.R.C.S.
Surgeon, Department of Gastro-enterology
Frenchay Hospital, Bristol
Clinical Lecturer in Surgery
University of Bristol

Wolfe Medical Publications Ltd
Year Book Medical Publishers, Inc.

Published by Wolfe Medical Publications 1987
Printed by W.S. Cowell Ltd, 8 Buttermarket, Ipswich, England

ISBN 0 7234 0832 7

This book is one of the titles in the series of Wolfe Medical Atlases, a series which brings together probably the world's largest systematic published collection of diagnostic colour photographs.
For a full list of Atlases in the series, plus forthcoming titles and details of our surgical, dental and veterinary Atlases, please write to Wolfe Medical Publications Ltd, Wolfe House, 3 Conway Street, London W1P 6HE.
or
Year Book Medical Publishers, Inc,
35 East Wacker Drive, Chicago, Ill. 60601

General Editor, Wolfe Medical Atlases:
G. Barry Carruthers, MD(London)

Distributed in Continental North and Central America, Hawaii and Puerto Rico by Year Book Medical Publishers, Inc.

Library of Congress Cataloging in Publication Data

Celestin, L. R.
A colour atlas of the surgery and management of intestinal stomas.
Includes bibliographies and index.
1. Enterostomy—Atlases. I. Title. [DNLM:
1. Colostomy—atlases. 2. Ileostomy—atlases.
WI 17 C392c]
RD540.6.C36 1986 617'.554 85-10910
ISBN 0-8151-1484-2

CONTENTS

Foreword 6

Acknowledgements 6

Preface 7

Milestones in Stomatherapy 8

Section I: General principles 11

Chapter I: Types of stoma and their physiology 12

II: Indications and Pathology 16

III: Constructing the stoma
Part I: Choosing the site 29
Part II: Preparing the site 34

IV: Constructing the spout 39

V: The muco-cutaneous suture 42

VI: Choice of appliance 45

VII: The transverse colostomy 49

VIII: The ileostomy effluent 54

IX: The perineal wound 55

X: The abdominal incision 63

XI: Some abnormal stomas 66

Section II: Complications 73

XII: Poor siting 74

XIII: Stoma proper 78

XIV: Muco-cutaneous junction 88

XV: Skin problems 99

XVI: Peristomal skin (including skin under plate) 101

XVII: The skin under the pouch 107

XVIII: The peri-intestinal area 108

Section III: Appliances and accessories 115

Appendix 128

Useful addresses 137

Index 138

FOREWORD

This work would have been inconceivable in the early days of my surgical career forty years ago – and not just because the elegant form of presentation which Wolfe Publications has mastered had yet to be developed. At that time colostomy was virtually the sole form of intestinal excretory stoma and although the operation had been undertaken in one way or other for centuries the patients and those who looked after them had remained content with the rather cumbersome forms of appliance, or even simple dressings, which had been their lot virtually since 1824 when Maitland and his bookkeeper patient, Baron, experimented with trusses, tin boxes and sponges in order to create a device for colostomy control. Here, in principle at least, was an attempt to control excreta; but the principle had to be abandoned in favour of regulating excretion by ensuring that each day began with evacuation of the bowel in the hope that no soiling would occur until further evacuation at a propitious moment at the end of the day, or again next morning. To obtain this desirable end much discussion surrounded the appropriate diet to be ingested and the regular habits to be inculcated on the one hand, or the more drastic approach of a daily bowel washout on the other. The pros and cons made useful contributions to articles but there was never enough to fill a book. Furthermore the underlying attitude to colostomy was negative; the concept of stoma care in a positive sense as we know it today was yet to come.

Fortunately history repeated itself though the scene shifted from Blackburn, England, where Maitland had practised, to Chicago, USA. There in 1944 Strauss persuaded Koenig, a chemistry student in whom he had undertaken ileostomy and colectomy, to design a leak-proof appliance. The outcome was an adherent bag, which was marketed by Rutzen. The control of excreta was back in favour, and none too soon since this could provide the only solution to the problems posed by the fluid, erosive and uncontrollable effluent from an ileostomy.

The Koenig/Rutzen bag opened many doors: to surgery for ulcerative colitis: to the use of ileum in a urinary conduit: to stoma clinics and stoma care. These advances brought benefits to colostomy patients in their train.

Art and science acquire their own literature; there is an art and science of stoma care, here appropriately presented by a surgeon since the conduct of surgery invokes both art and science. Both are manifest in this presentation; also in the solutions Mr Celestin advocates and demonstrates for the problems inherent in this field, culled from his wide experience.

Bryan N Brooke. MD, MChir, FRCS, Hon FRACS.

ACKNOWLEDGEMENTS

I wish to acknowledge all those who have assisted me in the preparation of this book.

First and foremost the many patients who have allowed me to photograph them and so made this atlas possible.

Those colleagues, too numerous to list, who have referred me patients with various stomal problems requiring rectification or advice; or who have provided me with examples of stomal conditions that have allowed me to make the atlas as complete as possible. I am specially grateful to Mr. R. G. Finemore and Mr. I. D. Hunter-Craig; Professor Robin Williamson; Mr. W. F. W. Southwood; Dr. R. Sultan; Mr. R. E. May; Dr. Richard Harvey and Dr. Nassif Ibrahim.

I have received invaluable help, and indeed guidance, from our Departmental Stomatherapist and Senior Nursing Officer Mr. A. Helmore whose care of my patients has been unstinting, and many of the excellent results depicted in this book have been his work.

Much of the photography was done during operations. I am grateful to the operating theatres Nursing Staff, my Anaesthetic colleagues and my Junior Staff for their patience with me while this was being done.

My greatest thanks go to the Department of Medical Photography and Illustration of Frenchay Hospital. Over the years they have generously given of their time and efforts and have contributed substantially to this work, most specially Mr. Simon Tutty and Mr. Pete Cox.

I received invaluable help from most Appliance Suppliers which provided me either with perfect samples for photography or with actual photographs – some historical – of appliances as well as of unusual clinical problems. I have greatly appreciated their contribution.

L. R. Celestin

PREFACE

Social evolution, with its accent on hygiene, has moved people further and further away from their primitive ways to a life of obsessive control over their sphincters, with some form of revulsion against all body wastes and smells. As the infant progresses to adulthood, this concept of cleanliness is impressed upon him. Destruction of sphincters safeguarding this image is a traumatic experience, and adjustment can only be achieved if the patient receives, at all levels, that quality of management which is possible only if the highest degree of technical ability and compassion are displayed.

Thus the patient will judge the success of a procto-colectomy or of an abdomino-perineal excision of the rectum on three main features of the operation.

Foremost will be the stoma. A trouble-free one is a boon. A troublesome one can bring about social, domestic and psychological upsets. It is therefore imperative that it should be constructed with demanding care, and its proper siting should be the first step of any operation.

Next comes the perineal wound. One that heals by first intention will speed up the patient's recovery and boost his or her morale. If it cavitates or breaks down, it may be months or even years before healing finally takes place; and the resulting fibrosis could cause recurrent discomfort.

Finally, an abdominal wound that heals without complication will make the wearing of an appliance easier and will do away with the additional grief caused by an unsightly scar.

The hallmark of success on all three scores rests with meticulous and exacting surgical technique. Attention to details; operating time spent on achieving a high standard; thorough pre-operative preparation of the patient with special reference to the nutritional status will be repaid time and again later on by gratifying results and above all by a grateful patient.

It is about the do's and don'ts of stoma surgery and management that this atlas is concerned, and it will endeavour to draw attention to various surgical techniques that have proved consistently reliable and rewarding. It is not intended to be an exhaustive work and is not meant to be a treatise on stoma care, which has already been very well covered in many excellent books. Its aim is simply to cover the everyday aspect of stoma management in as practical and visual a way as possible. In this context, it will not deal in detail with such new and sophisticated procedures as continent reservoirs and appliances, nor with the subjective aspects of stoma care.

Surgery will reach its noontide best when it will find means of eliminating the stoma. Its finest hour to date was when the eversion technique with its muco-cutaneous suture was introduced. The best judge of a book on stomas must be the very person whose efforts brought about this technique. I have therefore thought it appropriate to ask Prof. Bryan Brooke to write its foreword, and in so doing I am very conscious of the signal honour he has done me.

L. R. Celestin
Bristol 1986

MILESTONES IN STOMATHERAPY

PRAXAGORAS, 4th century B.C., probably performed the first bowel decompression by carrying out a colotomy, which he closed after having emptied the bowel of its contents.

1710 *Alexis LITTRÉ* (France) suggested the idea of a trans-peritoneal colostomy in the left iliac fossa as treatment for anal atresia. It followed observations he had made at the autopsy of a 6-day old baby who died from the complications of rectal atresia. The idea was not received with great enthusiasm by the Académie Royale des Sciences.

1776 *H. PILLORÉ* (France) performed the first elective caecostomy to relieve total obstruction from a rectal carcinoma. Progressive meteorism at the time was treated – as a desperate act – by trocar decompression of the over-distended bowel. Faecal peritonitis was frequent. But before resorting to this, obstructed colonic cancer was treated by the ingestion of up to a kilo of mercury. Pilloré's patient unfortunately died of this treatment, having developed gangrene of a loop of small bowel weighed down by the mercury.

1793 *C. DURET* (France) carried out the first successful elective ilio-lumbar colostomy kept exteriorised by suturing the meso-colon to the skin. The patient, a baby with an imperforate anus, lived to be 45.

1797 *Pierre FINE* (Switzerland) carried out a transverse colostomy via a sub-umbilical midline incision in a woman with a totally obstructed sigmoid colon carcinoma, with good results. The patient who had extensive liver secondaries, died 28 days later of marasmus.

1839 *Jean Zuléma AMUSSAT* (France) reported 29 cases treated by colostomy, 21 for imperforate anus and eight adults with malignancy. Four babies and five adults survived. Amussat recognised peritonitis as the main cause of death and therefore proposed an extra-peritoneal route suggesting a descending colostomy via a left lumbar approach (see p. 10).

1850 *James LUKE* (England) fashioned the first sigmoid colostomy through a left pararectal opening. He was President of the College twice, in 1853 and 1862 (see p. 114).

1855 *Karl THIERSCH* (Germany) used a defunctioning transverse colostomy to protect a distal anastomosis. Unfortunately, his patient died of peritonitis.

1879 *T. SCHEDE* (Germany) produced the first double-barrel colostomy as a sequel to an extra-abdominal excision of a colonic tumour. The operation was later repeated and popularised by Johann von Mikulicz-Radecki in 1903. It was improved by the creation of a spur that was crushed to re-establish continuity.

1907 *William Ernest MILES* (England) modified and popularised Charles Mayo's operation of abdomino-perineal excision (1904) for rectal carcinoma, carrying out the two separate operations in a single stage. The operation was probably first elaborated by Jean Quénu in the 1850s.

1917 *J. P. LOCKHART-MUMMERY* (England) reviewing 50 colostomies he had performed gave the first advice on *STOMA CARE*. Later, in 1927, he recommended the principle of colonic irrigation.

1934 *M. KIRSCHNER* (Germany), Professor of Surgery at Heidelberg, described the combined approach to the one-stage operation. The lithotomy position still proved a drawback to ease of access.

1935 *KOENIG and RUTZEN* (USA), the first ileostomy bag.

1939 *O. V. LLOYD-DAVIES* (England) using a lowered position, the lithotomy-Trendelenberg, facilitated the one-stage combined operation performed by two surgeons synchronously.

1952 *B. BROOKE* (England) solved most of the complications of the ileal stoma by creating an ileal spout that was everted upon itself and 'matured' by immediate muco-cutaneous suturing. It opened a new era in stoma construction (see p. 36).

1958 *P. SAMES* (England, Bath, in March) and *J. C. GOLIGHER* (England, Leeds, in September) described independently the technique of a retroperitoneal tunnel to prevent internal herniation in sigmoid colostomies.

1961 *R. B. TURNBULL* (USA) proposed stomatherapy as a new discipline and trained the first stomatherapist, Norma Gill. This was a major step in the professional care of the 'ostomate', until then left to the lay comfort of empathic societies (see p. 70).

1969 *N. G. KOCK* (Sweden) described an ileal reservoir to eliminate the use of an appliance in ileostomies. This was to open the way to efforts at the elimination of the stoma itself, a concept that found its strongest proponent in the late Sir Alan Parkes.

1975 *H. FEUSTEL and G. HERRING* (Germany) described the use of a magnetic ring and, magnetic cap as a means of producing a seal that would render 'continent' a colostomy.

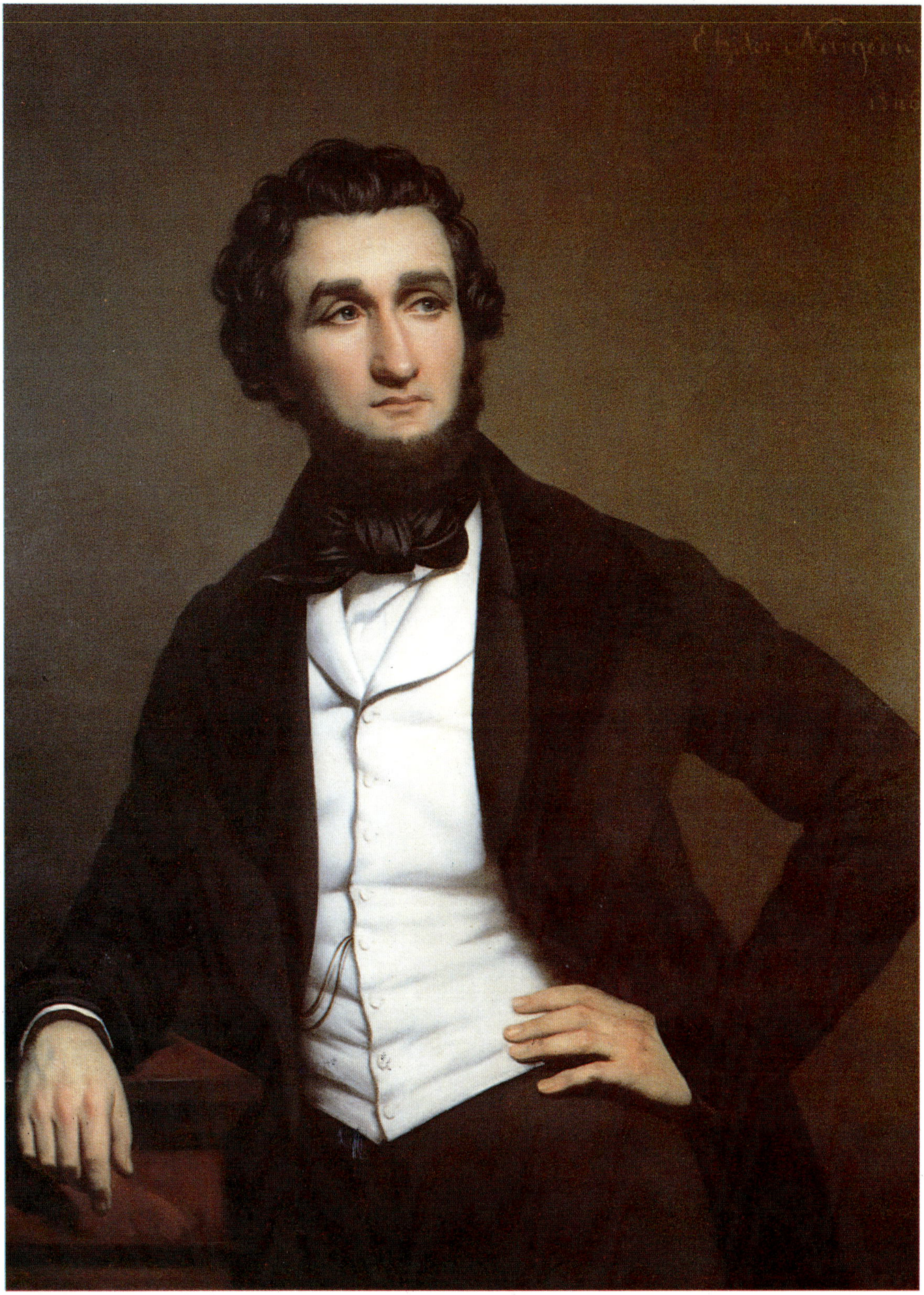

Jean Zuléma Amussat
(1796–1856)
Founder of Stoma Surgery
(By Courtesy of Wellcome Trustees)

Section I General Principles

I: TYPES OF STOMA AND THEIR PHYSIOLOGY

1

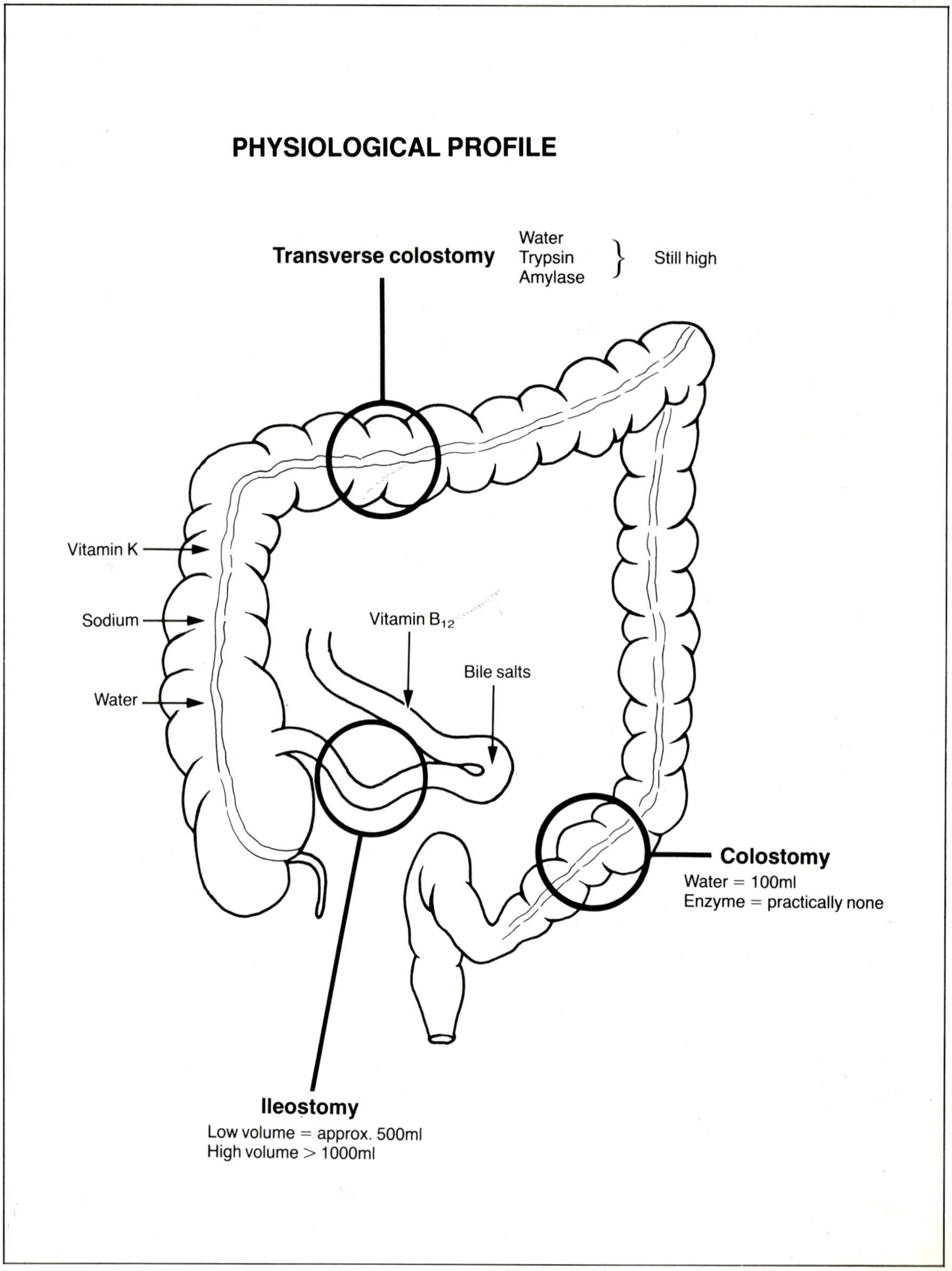

1 The profiles of the three commonest stomas are sketched here, with emphasis on the water, enzyme, vitamin and electrolyte content of their effluents.

2

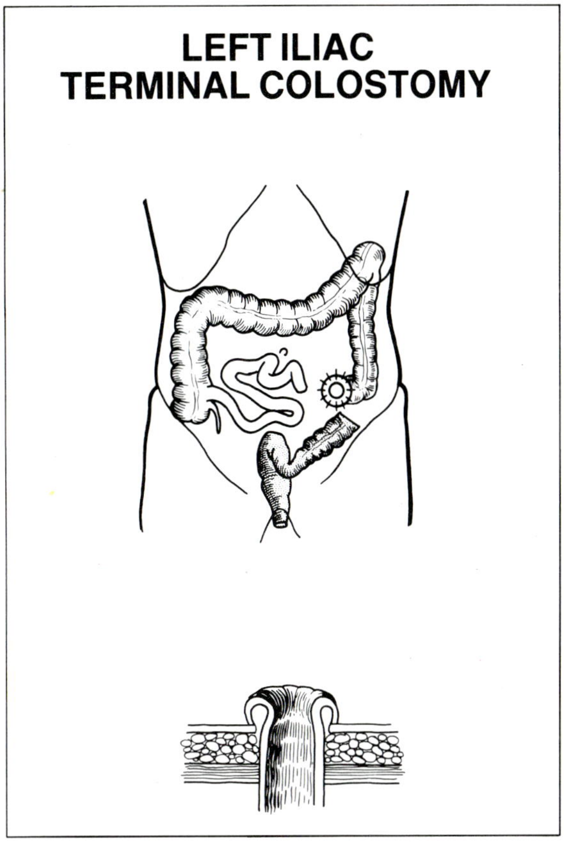

2 The commonest colostomy: the left iliac terminal. It presents a short everted spout, 1–2 cm tall.

3

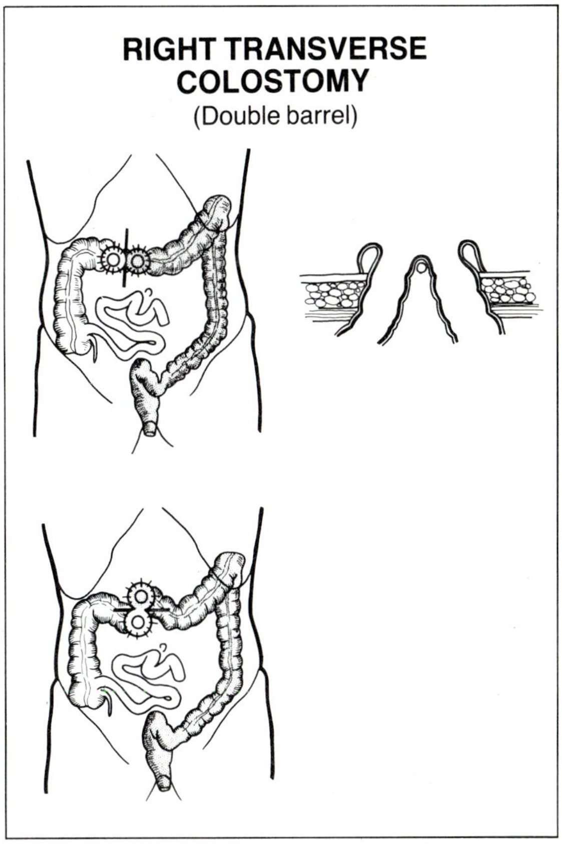

3 The right transverse colostomy is usually a 'defunctioning' one. It has two barrels kept exteriorised by a support. The barrels may lie in a horizontal or in a vertical plane.

4

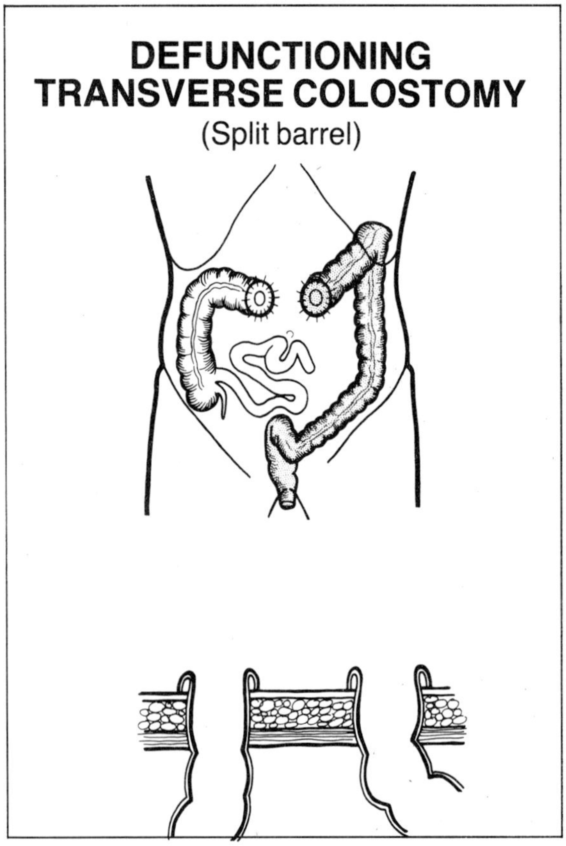

4 Complete defunctioning requires that the barrels of a transverse colostomy be split and separated; the distal one becoming a mucus fistula.

5

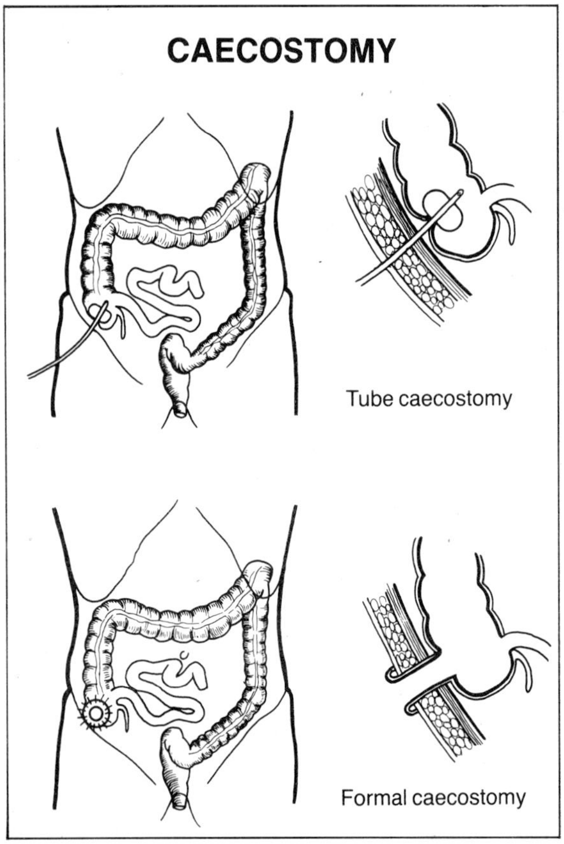

5 A caecostomy as a formal operation is almost obsolete, but a tube caecostomy is still used as a decompressing 'blow-hole', or as a safety valve to protect a difficult low anastomosis.

Useful Ileostomy Data

Chemistry of an established low volume ileostomy

	Concentration	Daily Loss
Water	—	± 500 ml
Sodium	115 mmol/l	55 ± 25 mmol
Potassium	8 mmol/l	4.5 ± 1 mmol
Chloride	45 mmol/l	20 ± 5 mmol
Calcium	25 mmol/l	12 ± 3 mmol
Phosphorus	—	150 mg
Bilirubin	—	70–100 mg
Trypsin	0.7 IU/ml	350 IU
Amylase	240 U/ml	120 000 U
pH	6.0–6.5	

Volume and wet weight

The ileostomy effluent is increased by some foods such as prune juice and cabbage.

The water output is not affected by a high water intake; but an intake of more than 15 g of sodium chloride a day will increase it.

Isogel increases the volume of the effluent and thickens it.

Diphenoxylate (Lomotil); loperamide (Imodium) and codeine phosphate all decrease the water output.

Na^+/K^+ ratio is normally 12:1, but in the early post-operative period and in conditions causing salt depletion it can fall as low as 2:1.

Bacteriology

The distal ileum becomes heavily colonised in an ileostomy. Anaerobes, aerobes and fungi all increase in number, the total population being at least a 100-fold larger than in the normal ileum. Coliforms show the highest increase, of up to 2000-fold.

Intestinal gases

A normal adult produces 500 ml of flatus/day: 30% methane, 60% N, O_2 & CO_2 in equilibrium with plasma levels. Most of the methane is of colonic origin.

An ileostomy patient produces less gas: 70% N; the rest is O_2, CO_2 and other gases.

The smell of ileostomy flatus comes from the bacterial breakdown of some foods, such as onion, cabbage, spices and fish; and is due to methane, hydrogen sulphide and mercaptans.

An aspirin tablet dropped in a pouch is an effective deodorant. Oral chlorophyll and bismuth subgallate have proved useful in controlling a persistent odour of intestinal origin.

6
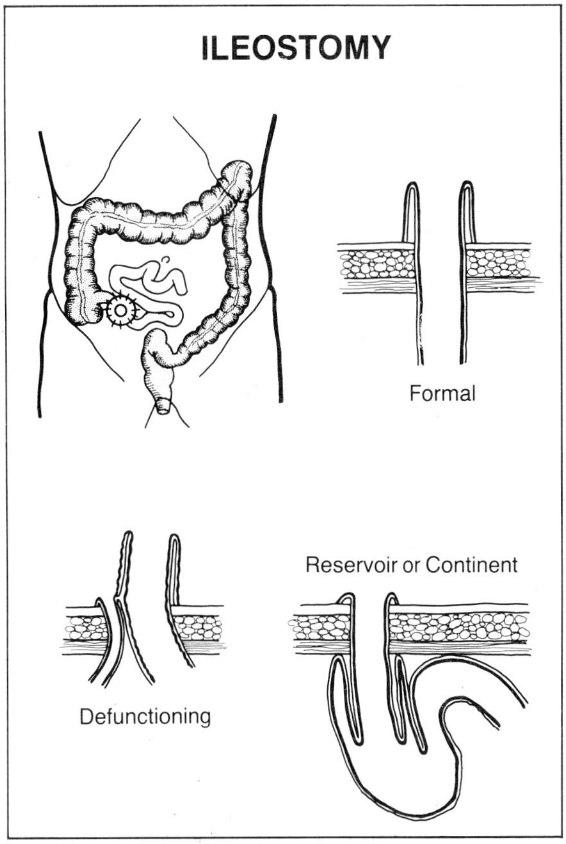

6 There are several varieties of ileostomy, of which the formal or right iliac terminal one is the commonest. It should have a spout of 2–3 cm, as should also the defunctioning variety. By contrast, the reservoir type needs only a flush stoma.

II: INDICATIONS AND PATHOLOGY

Indications

Colostomy

A. *Cancer of the rectum and anus; rare carcinoid tumours of the rectum*

(a) *Palliative* and/or *Defunctioning:*
– in irresectable lesions.
– in recto-vaginal or recto-vesical fistulae.
– as an adjunct to radiotherapy.

(b) *Curative:* – abdomino-perineal excision of anus and rectum.

(c) *Temporary:* – in Hartmann's procedure.
– gross dilatation in obstructive lesions.

All three types may overlap, in that tumours may become resectable after defunctioning or radiotherapy; or found to be inoperable after a colostomy planned to be temporary.

B. *Inflammatory lesions of the colon and rectum*

(a) *Complications of diverticulitis:*
– perforation.
– obstruction.
– abscess formation and fistulae.
– uncontrollable haemorrhage (rare).

(b) *Ulcerative proctitis* (rare).

(c) *Rectal and anal Crohn's disease with fistulae.*

In such cases the colostomy can be temporary or permanent, loop or terminal.

C. *As a protective measure*

When dehiscence of an anastomosis is feared (sometimes performed as a caecostomy).

D. *Less commonly in:*

(a) Traumatic lesions of the colon or rectum.

(b) Post-irradiation proctitis.

(c) Ischaemic colitis.

(d) Invasive endometriosis.

(e) Congenital conditions, e.g. Hirschsprung's disease.

(f) Sigmoid volvulus in patients too ill for major surgery.

(g) Total cord damage above sacral outflow, to facilitate nursing.

Ileostomy

This may be permanent or temporary. Permanent ones are fashioned in all conditions requiring a procto-colectomy. The main indications for permanent ones are:

A. *Inflammatory diseases,* mainly

(a) Ulcerative colitis and its complications.

(b) Extensive and severe Crohn's disease of the colon.

B. *Precancerous and cancerous conditions*

(a) Familial polyposis.

(b) Multiple colonic cancer.

Temporary ileostomies are usually a protective measure or may be defunctioning. They find a place in:

(a) Uncontrollable low intestinal fistulae.

(b) Right colonic trauma.

(c) To protect an anastomosis, usually an ileorectal one.

(d) Rare cases of congenital extrophy of the bladder and caecum.

(e) As a first stage of an ileo-anal reservoir.

Pathology

Carcinoma of the rectum

7

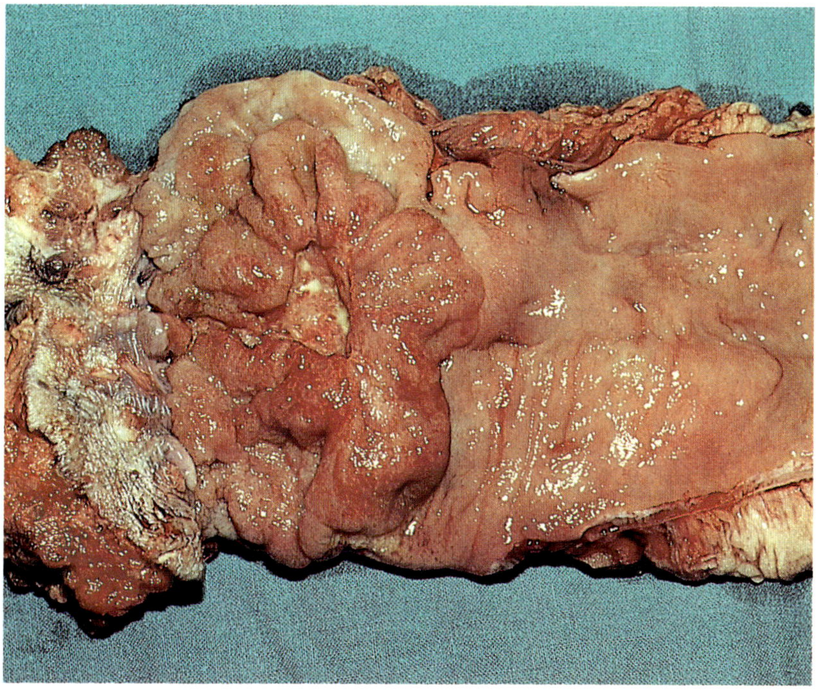

7 An ulcerating carcinoma of the rectum close to the anal verge. It was treated by an abdomino-perineal excision of the anus and rectum.

8

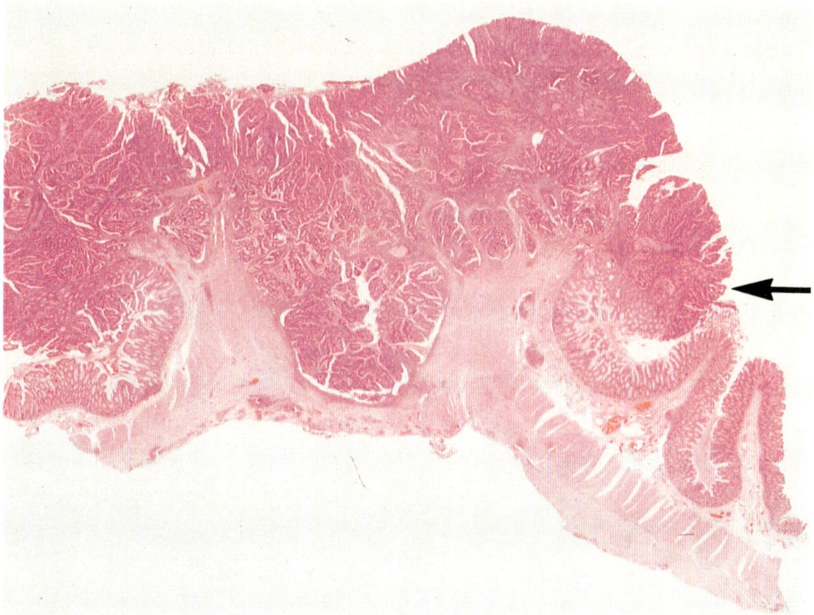

8 Low power microscopy of a typical adenocarcinoma. The sudden change (arrowed) from the pale cells of the normal glands to the darkly staining ones of the neoplastic area is very obvious. The normal glandular formation is lost, the muscularis mucosae has been destroyed, the muscle coat has been infiltrated, and there is a marked stromal reaction.

Polyposis coli

9

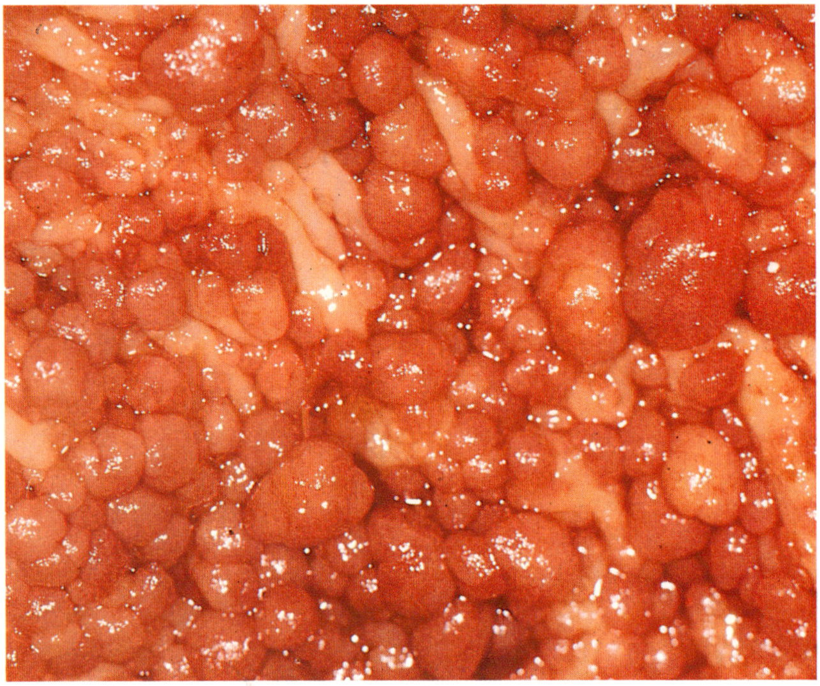

9 Familial polyposis treated by a procto-colectomy. Part of the sigmoid colon.

10

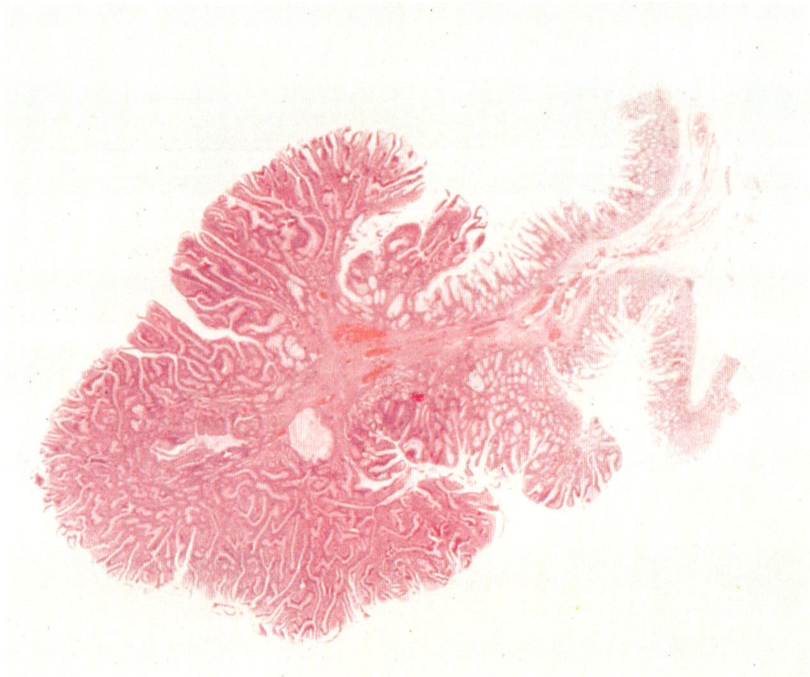

10 Low power microscopy of a polyp. It has branching fronds and tubules – typical of a tubovillous adenoma, which accounts for almost a third of all polyps. An intact muscularis mucosae lines the stalk in close proximity to the epithelial elements. When malignancy supervenes, the muscularis mucosae is disrupted by invading malignant cells. Ulceration later destroys the polyp totally.

11

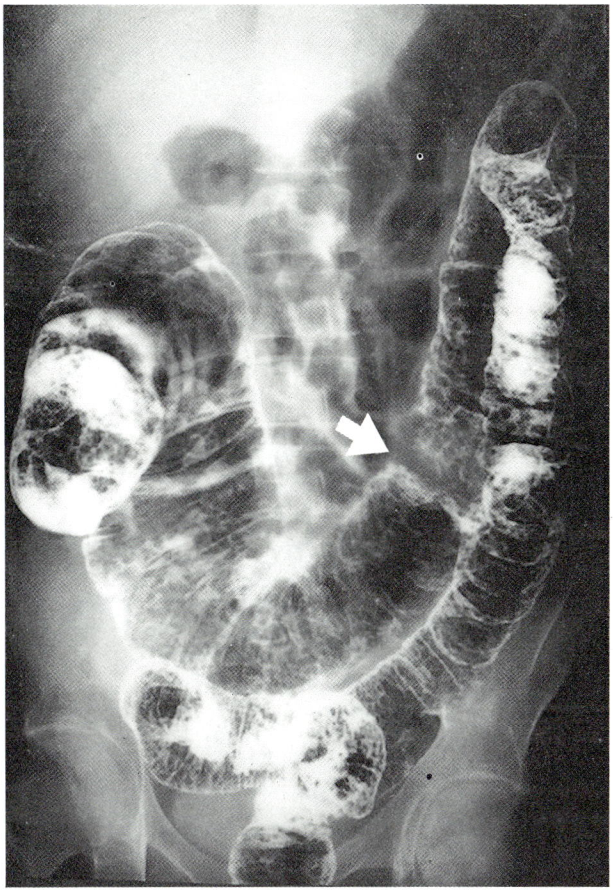

11 Barium enema: Polyposis coli complicated by malignancy in the left half of the transverse colon (arrowed). This was a familial case that escaped the tracing procedure.

12

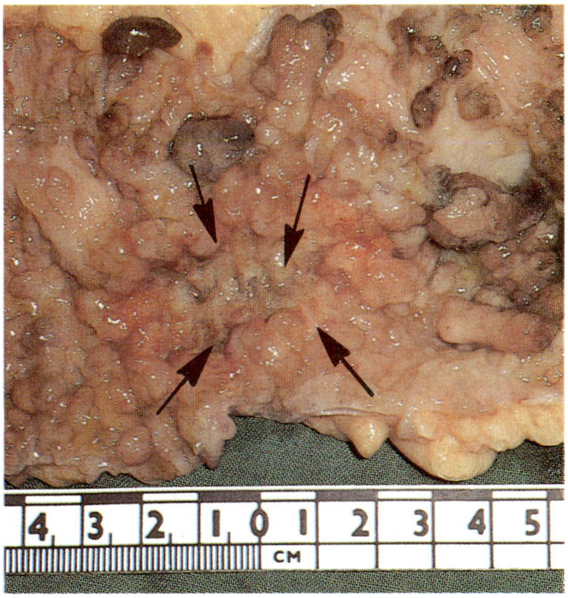

12 Macroscopical appearance. At the site of malignancy (arrowed) on the mesenteric border of the transverse colon, an ulcerated area has replaced the polyps and led to narrowing of the lumen, as is well shown in the radiological picture above.

13

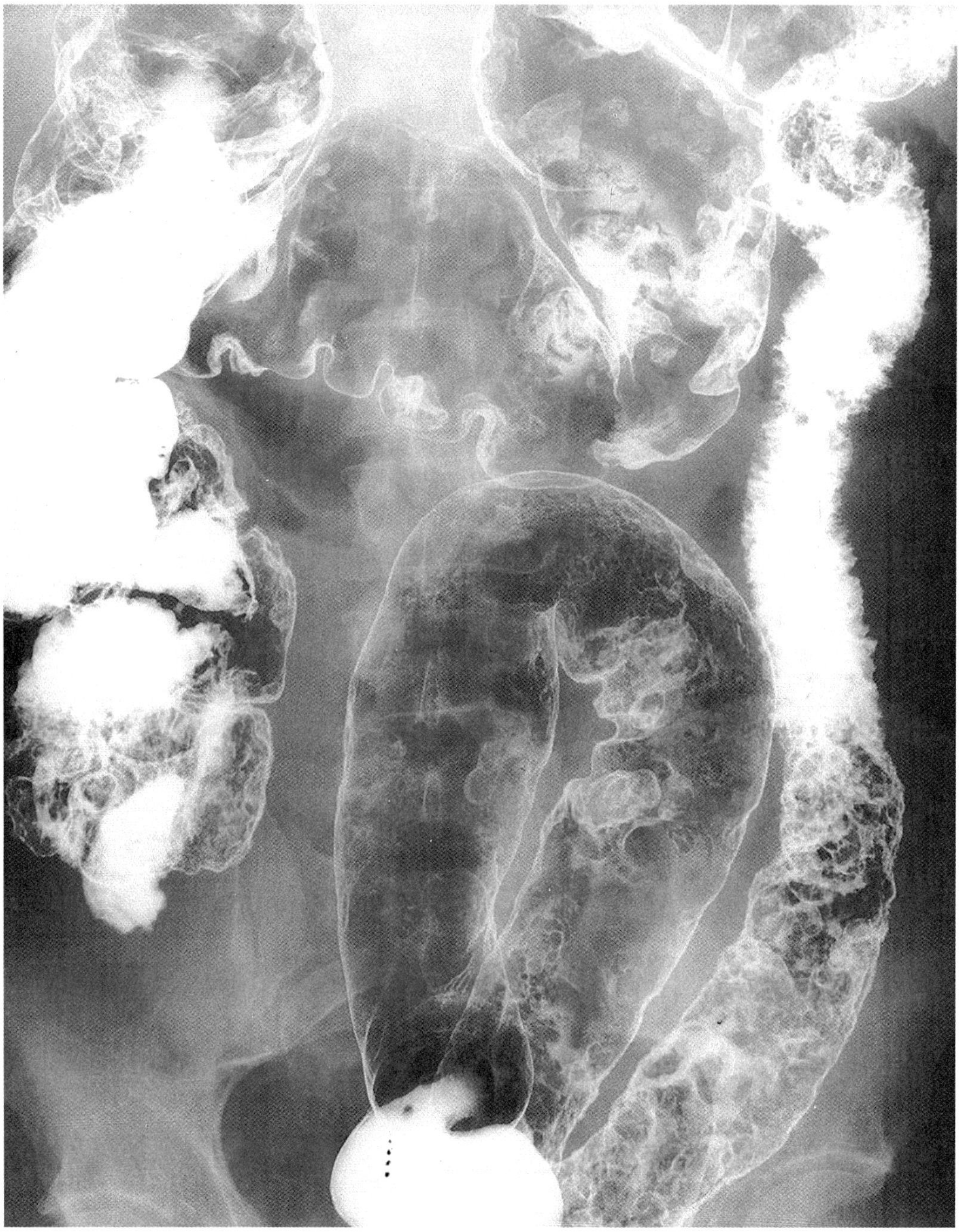

13 A case of acquired non-familial polyposis.

Patients present with diarrhoea that may be bloody and mimic ulcerative colitis. The Barium enema may show polyposis and areas of ulceration. This is the Cronkhite-Canada syndrome. It is a protein-losing enteropathy more in need of nutritional support than radical surgery. Alopecia and hyperpigmentation are other presenting symptoms.

Investigate the rest of the G.I. tract and examine a complete polyp.

14 Same case.

A Barium meal confirms large gastric polyps. More were found in the small bowel.

14

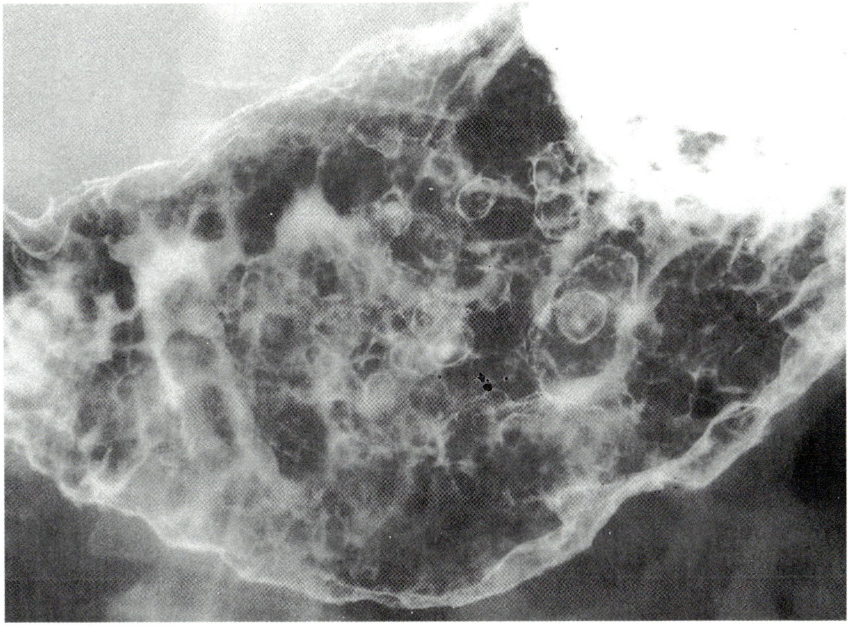

15

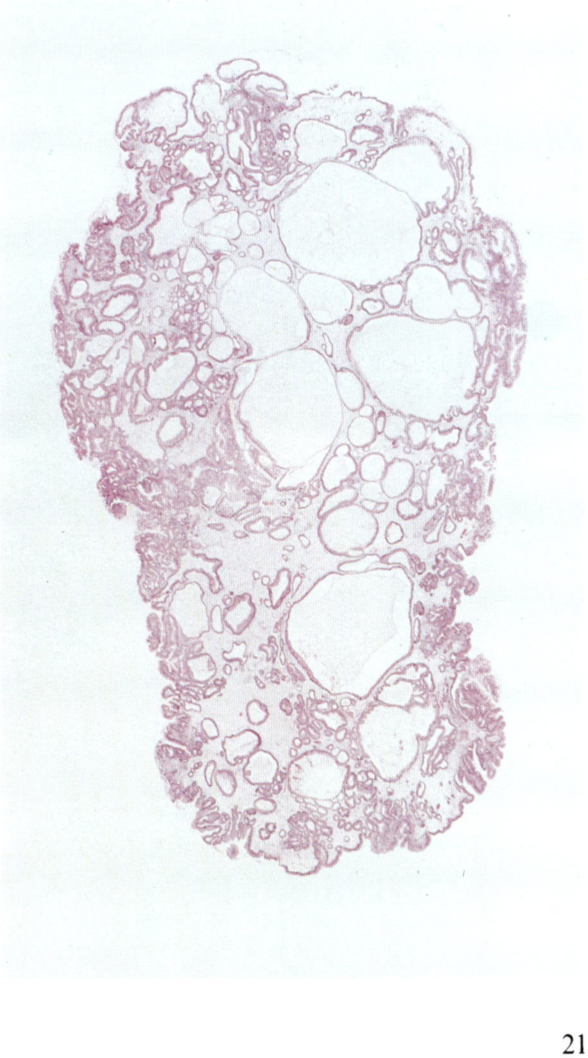

15 Low power section of a whole polyp from the same patient. It shows a cystic retention-type polyp and not an adenoma. Microscopy revealed inflammatory elements.

(Note that coincidental adenomatous polyps and carcinoma may be present.)

16

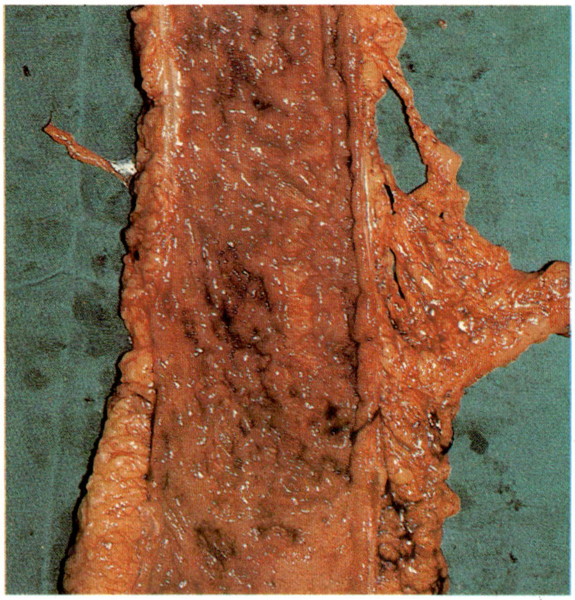

16 Ulcerative colitis involving the whole colon and rectum. Superficial ulcers several cm long, involving only the mucosa, are visible. The intervening mucosal bridges are oedematous giving a polypoidal-like effect (pseudo-polyps). Treated by procto-colectomy.

17

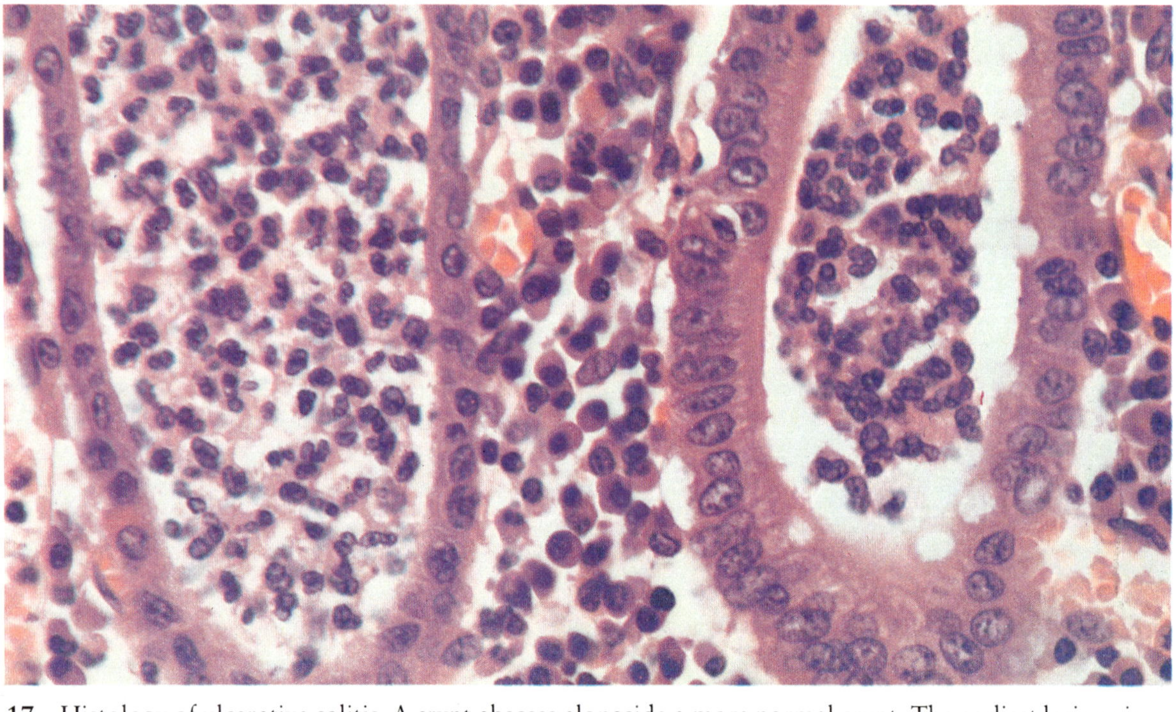

17 Histology of ulcerative colitis. A crypt abscess alongside a more normal crypt. The earliest lesions in ulcerative colitis are to be found in the crypts of the mucosal glands. Micro-abscesses appear and coalesce, undermining the mucosa which until then may have appeared normal. Mucosal necrosis follows, uncovering small flask shaped ulcers.

18

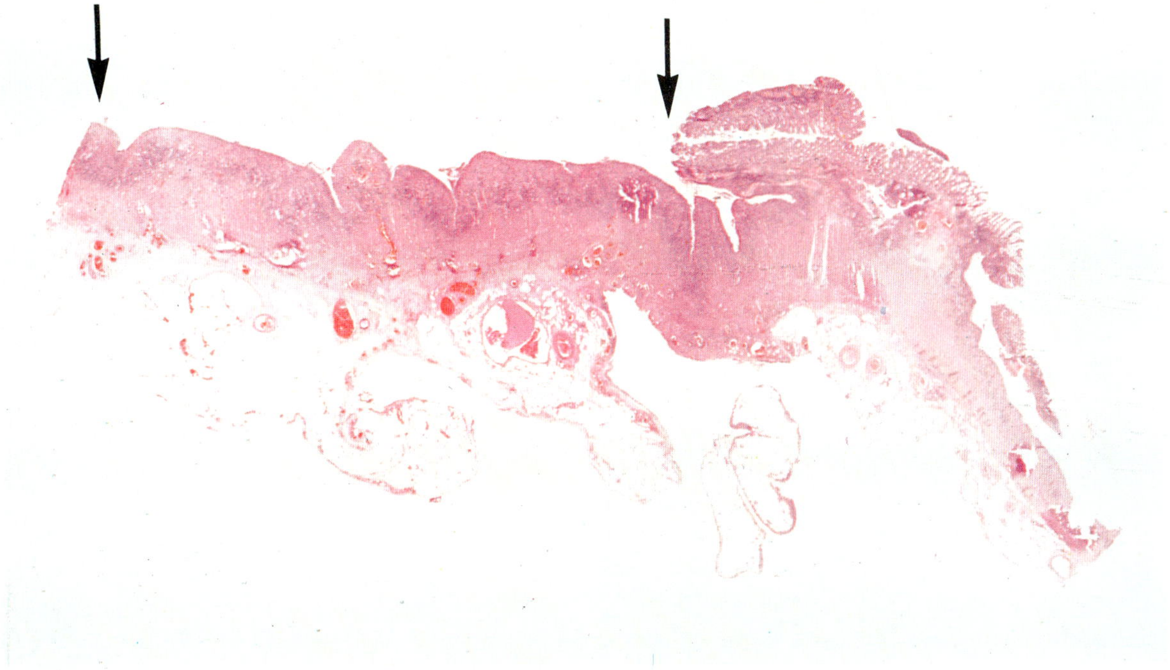

18 Low power microscopy of ulcerative colitis. As these ulcers extend, more mucosa sloughs (arrowed) leaving wide defects. These either border normal epithelium that bridges the defects or surround islands of normal looking epithelium which appear elevated in contrast, creating the polypoidal effect shown in **16** (above).

Note that the lesion in this type of colitis is essentially a mucosal one.

19

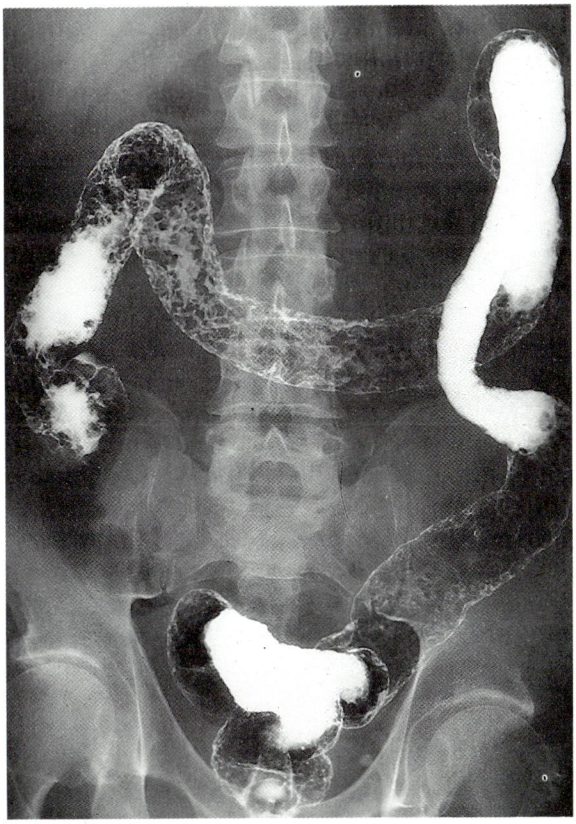

19 Barium enema in total proctocolitis.

Note the ribbon or tube-like outline due to loss of haustral pattern, with shortening of the colon and a granular appearance of the mucosa of the entire colon and rectum.

20

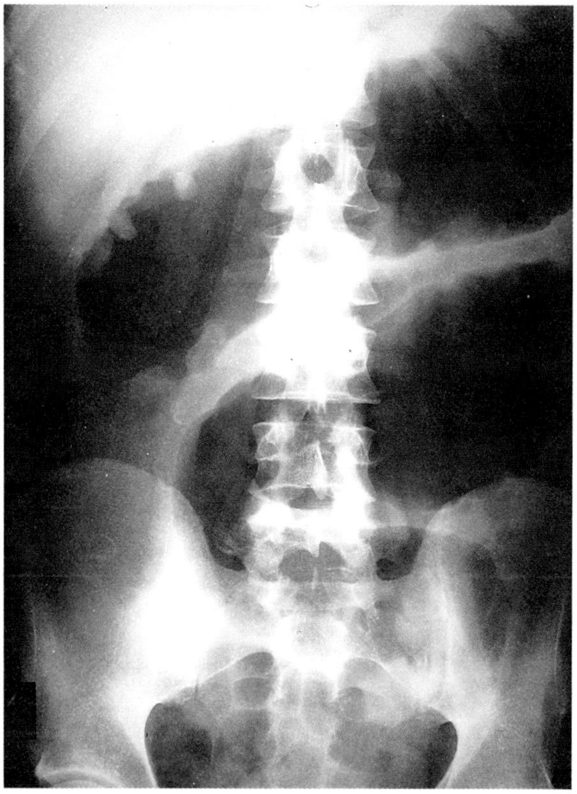

20 Acute fulminating ulcerative colitis: the toxic megacolon. Plain abdominal X-ray in the supine position showing gross dilatation of the colon, with well-outlined walls and mucosal remnants or islands (looking like polyps) projecting into the distended lumen.

The condition failed to respond to intensive medical treatment and required an urgent proctocolectomy.

21

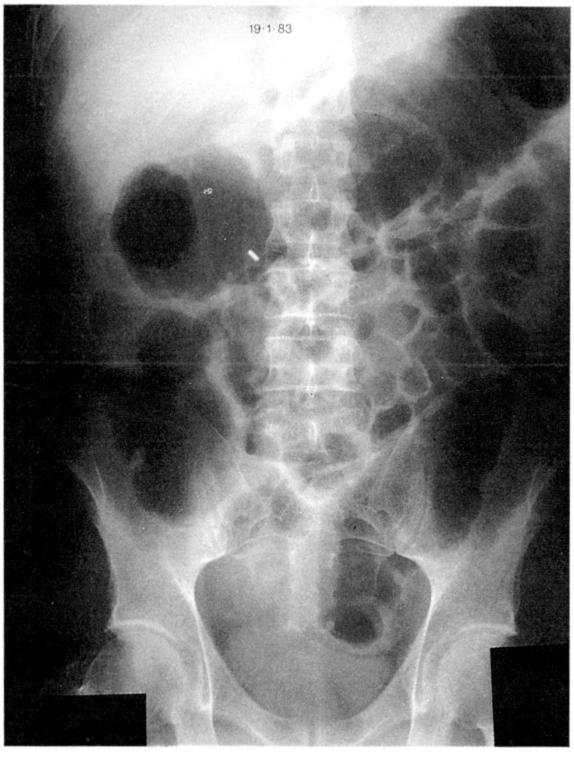

21 Radiograph of a patient with an early toxic megacolon. The ileo-caecal valve is incompetent and the distal small bowel is distended.

22

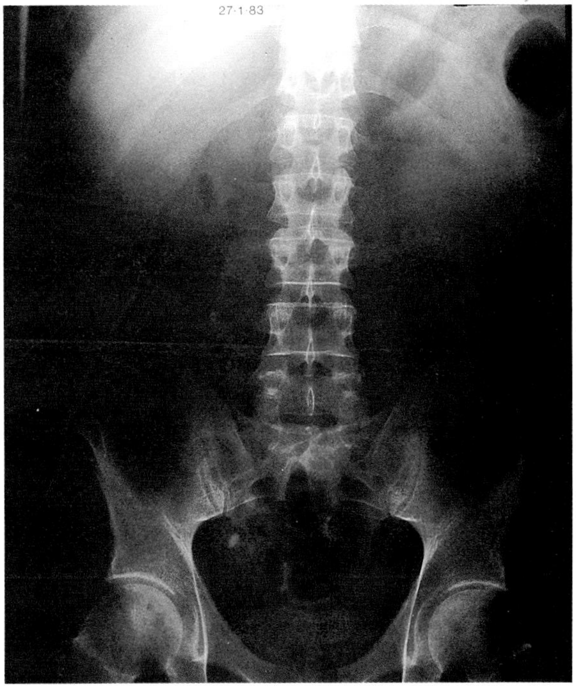

22 The same patient eight days after aggressive medical and nutritional treatment. The left colon is still slightly distended but later resolved.

23

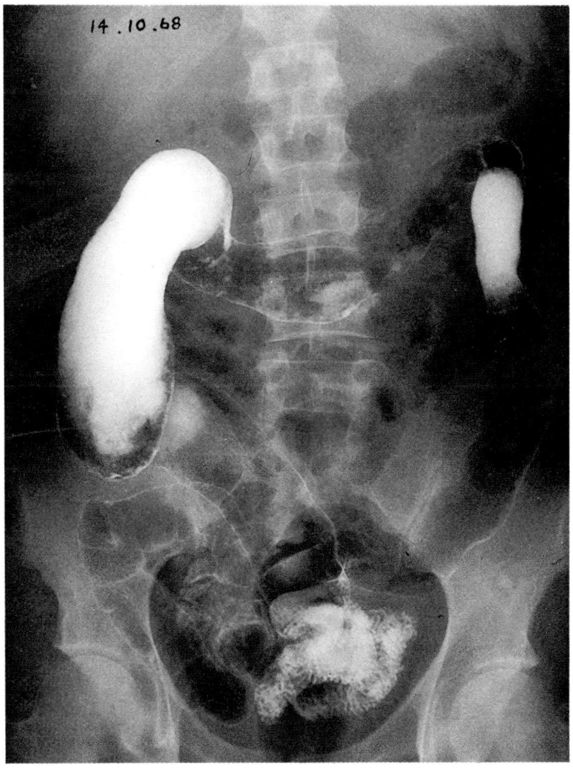

23 A long standing case of ulcerative colitis followed up at regular intervals. A sharp increase in plasma viscosity, without any change in symptoms, aroused suspicion and called for further barium studies (24).

24

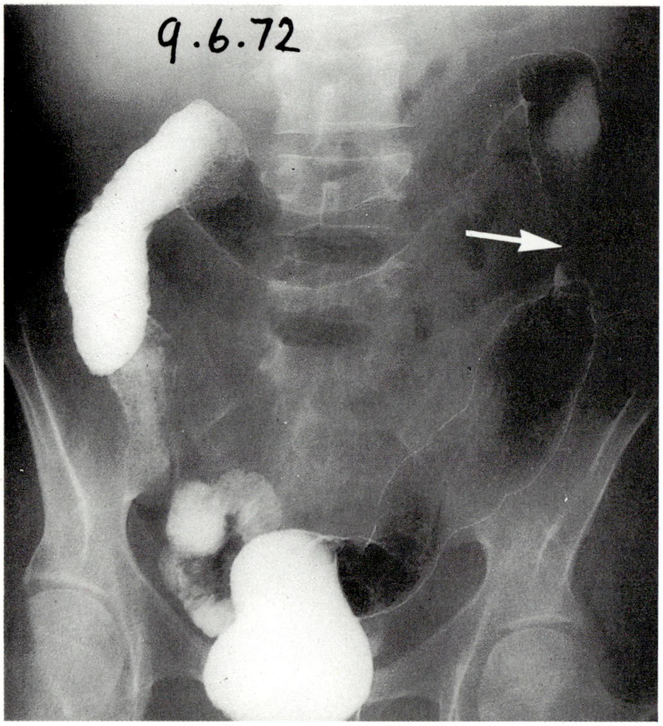

24 A carcinoma of the descending colon was clearly visible (arrowed).

25

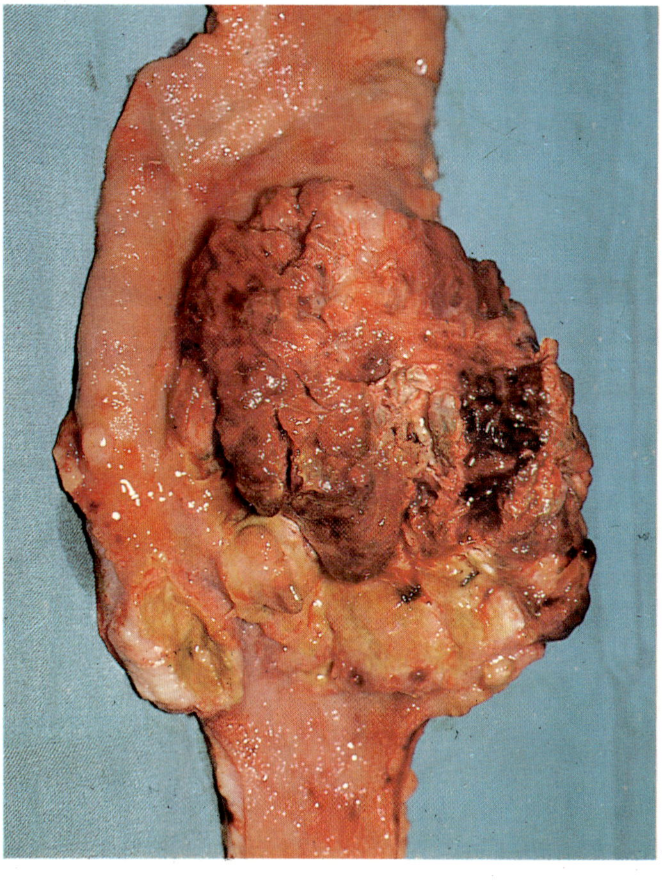

25 At procto-colectomy no distant spread was present though the lesion had encroached on most of the lumen.

26

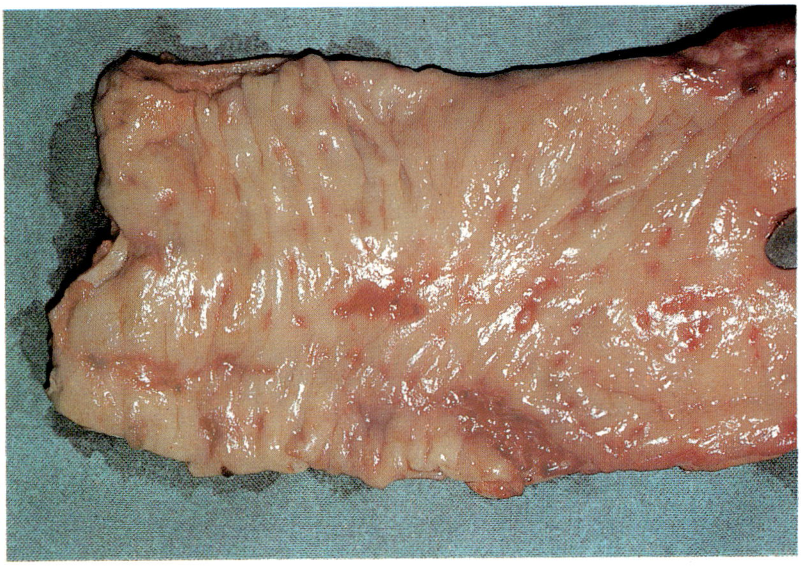

26 Total colonic Crohn's Disease sparing the small bowel.

Lesions in the transverse colon. Note the oedematous mucosa peppered with deep ulcers, many elongated or linear and lying in the long axis of the bowel; others coalescing.

27

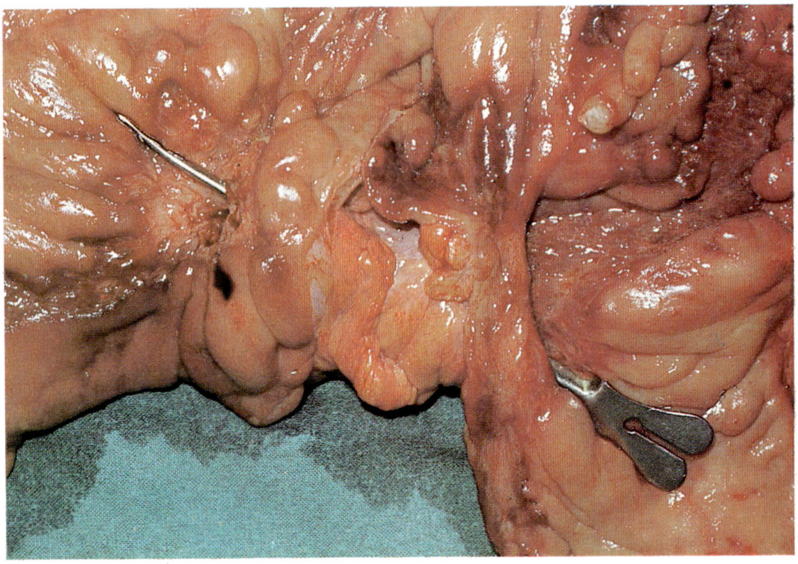

27 A colo-colic fistula in the same specimen at the splenic flexure. Deep ulcers have burrowed through the muscular coat and serosa with their channels joining up to form a fistulous tract.

28

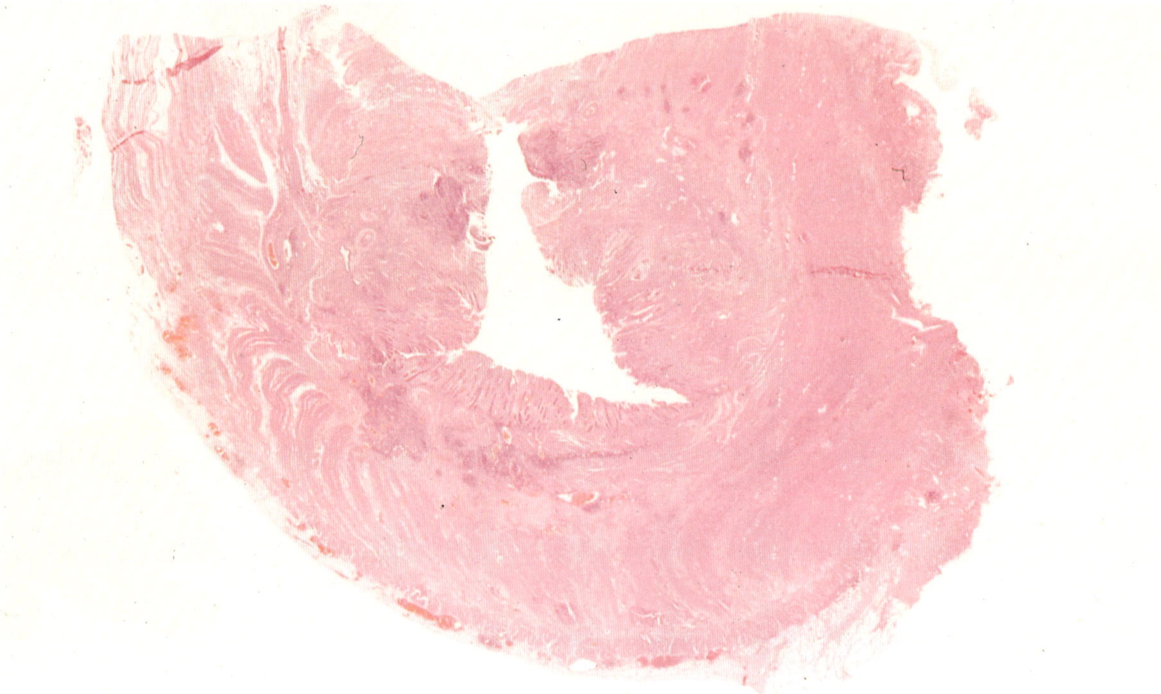

28 Crohn's colitis. In contrast to ulcerative colitis, the disease attacks the whole thickness of the bowel wall. Mucosal destruction is patchy. The submucosa is oedematous as the result of infiltration by inflammatory cells, and therefore encroaches upon the lumen. The muscularis mucosae is spared in places though the inflammatory reaction involves the muscular coat right down to the serosa, with marked thickening and fibrosis.

29

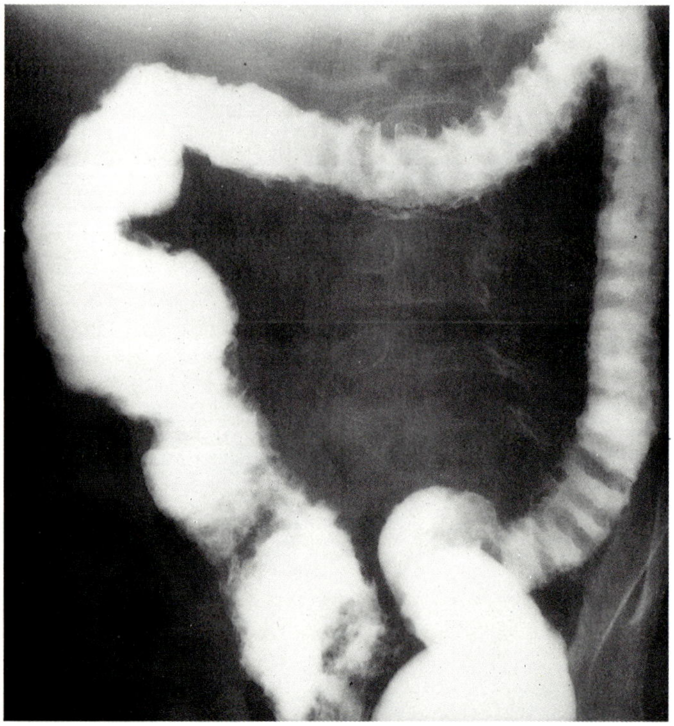

29 Radiograph of Crohn's colitis. The whole colon is involved. There is fissuring and deep undermining of the mucosa by ulceration and abscess formation, giving in parts a collar-stud profile. Note the typical cobblestone pattern of the mucosa.

III: CONSTRUCTING THE STOMA
PART I: CHOOSING THE SITE

Mark the site of the stoma carefully *before* the operation, avoiding skin creases, more so in obese patients. Check for absence of skin creases both in the lying and in the sitting position.

The umbilicus and the anterior superior iliac crest are the important landmarks in the proper siting of an ileostomy or an iliac colostomy; the right subcostal border and the umbilicus are the guides to a right transverse colostomy.

30

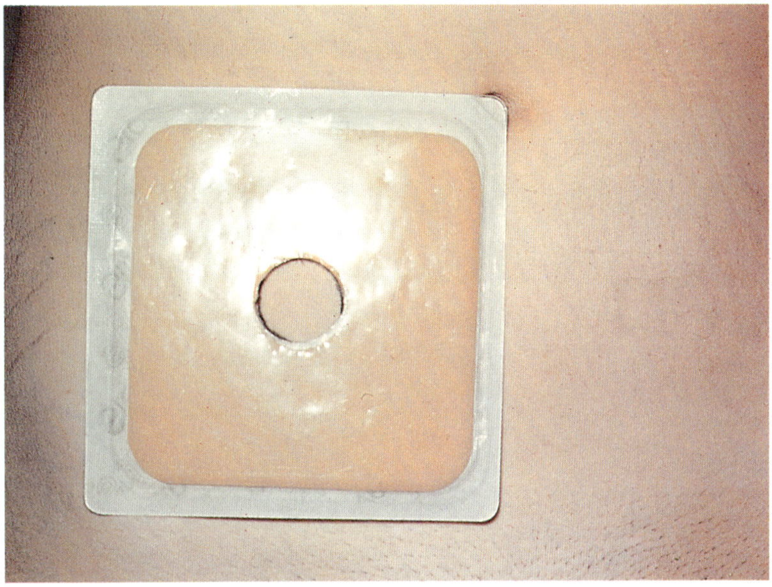

30 Site for an ileostomy. A stomahesive square with a centrally placed hole is an ideal template. One corner should be at the level of the umbilicus, and the diagonally opposite one should reach just short of the anterior superior iliac crest. Even in a thin patient this will be found useful – as here.

31

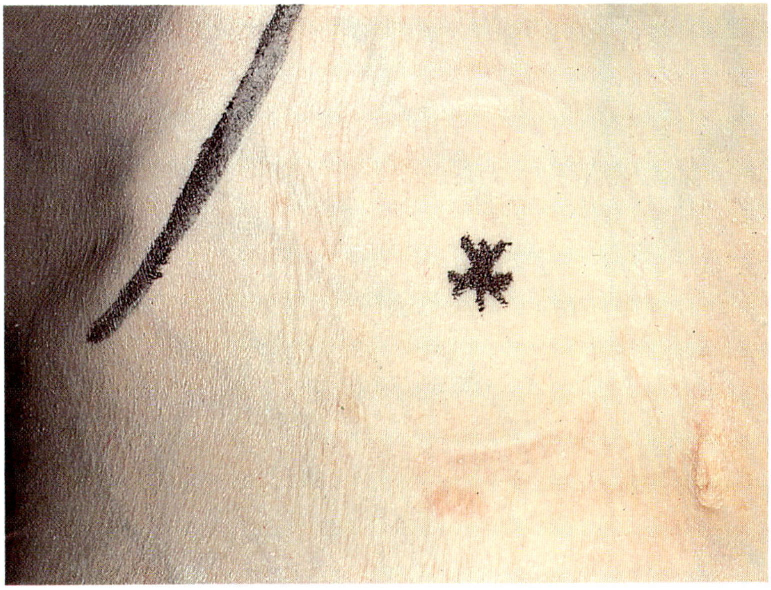

31 Site for a right transverse colostomy. Mark out the subcostal border, determining its nearest point to the umbilicus. The midposition between these two landmarks is the site of choice for a transverse colostomy.

32

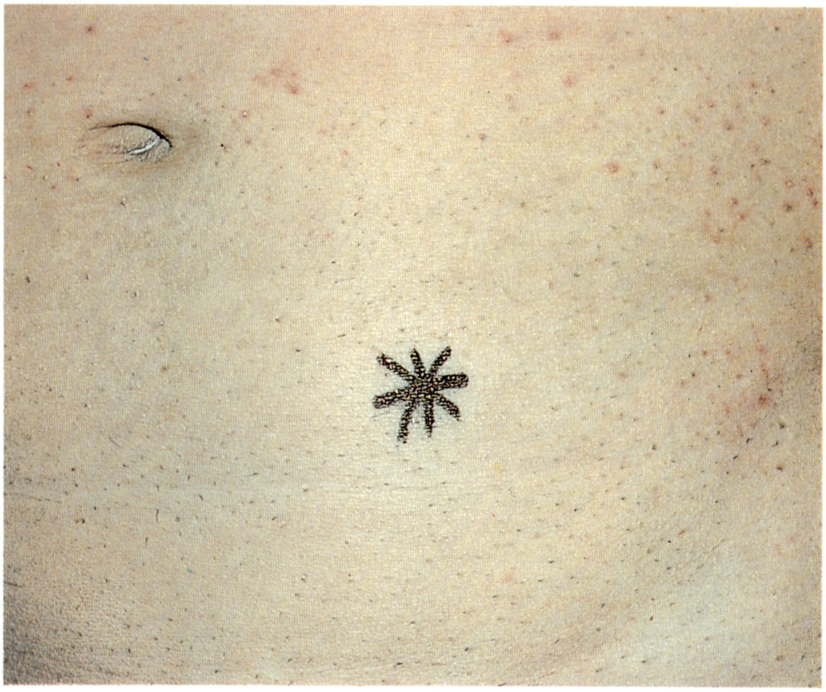

32 An obese patient in the supine position. The mark for a left iliac colostomy seems entirely acceptable.

33

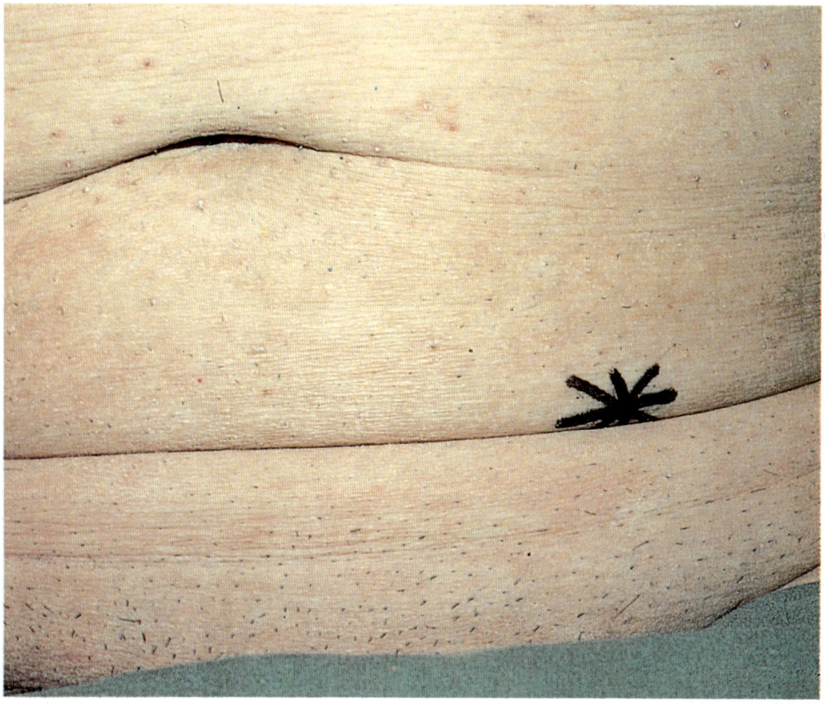

33 The same patient in the sitting position. A deep crease now crosses the lower aspect of the chosen site. This would interfere with the proper adherence of the plate and allow faeces to leak under the appliance.

34

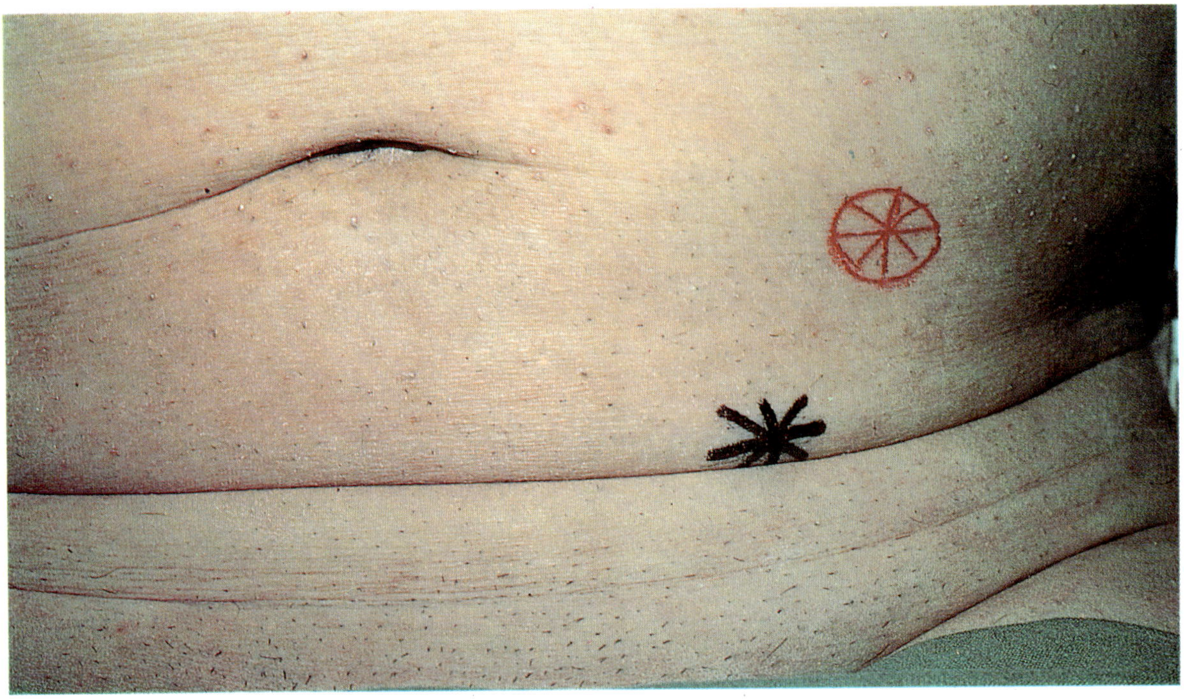

34 A site *away* from the crease must be chosen (marked in red) and the appliance tried and left *in situ* for a trial period before surgery.

35

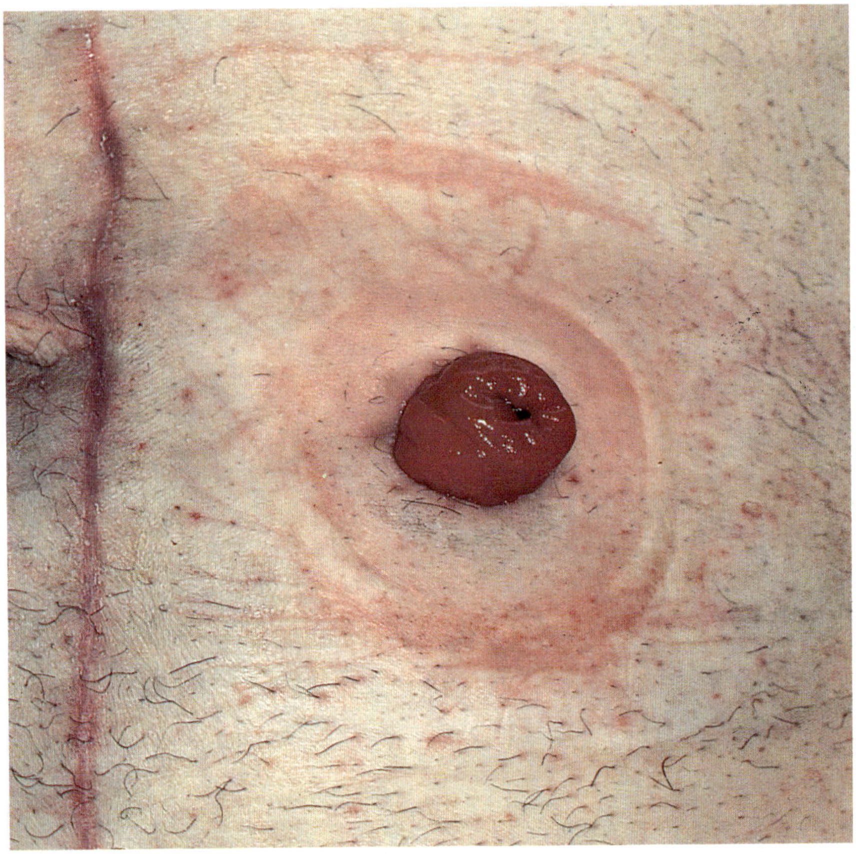

35 The same patient after surgery, with the stoma at the second site shown above. The appliance fits well, and does not overlap the abdominal incision despite being in a left paramedian position. This is usually the case in obese people.

36

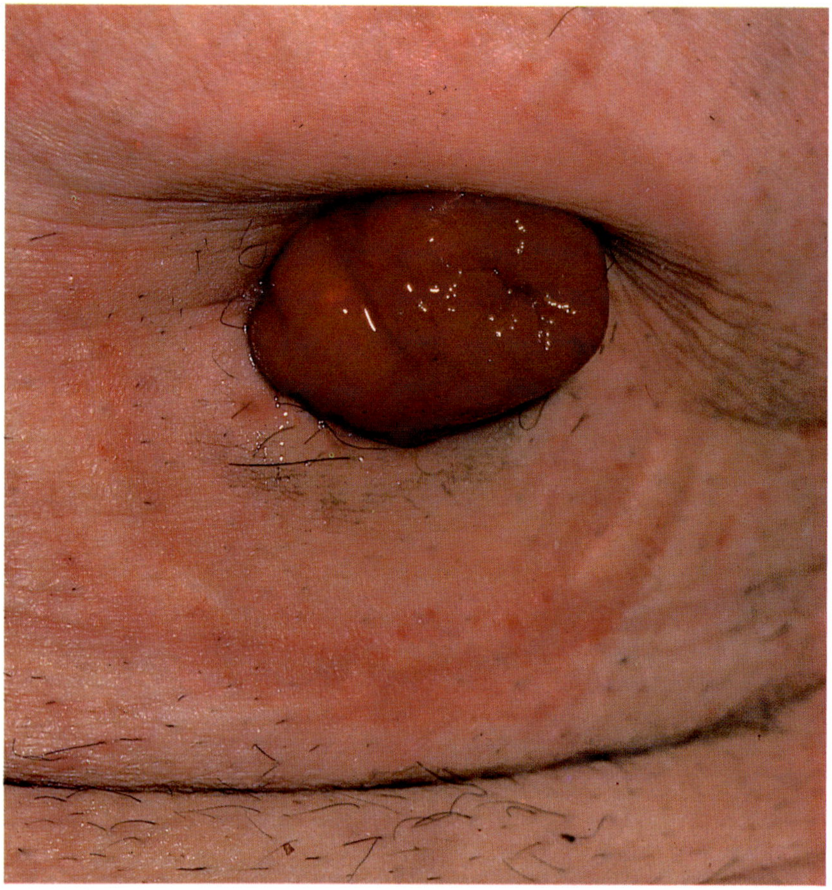

36 A patient in whom this simple precaution was not taken. Folds at the level of the colostomy, as well as above and below it, appear in the sitting position and hinder the fit of an appliance.

Having positioned the stoma carefully in relation to anatomical landmarks, incisions and drains should be sited so as not to interfere with the fitting of an appliance, as well as with articles of clothing such as belts, etc.

37

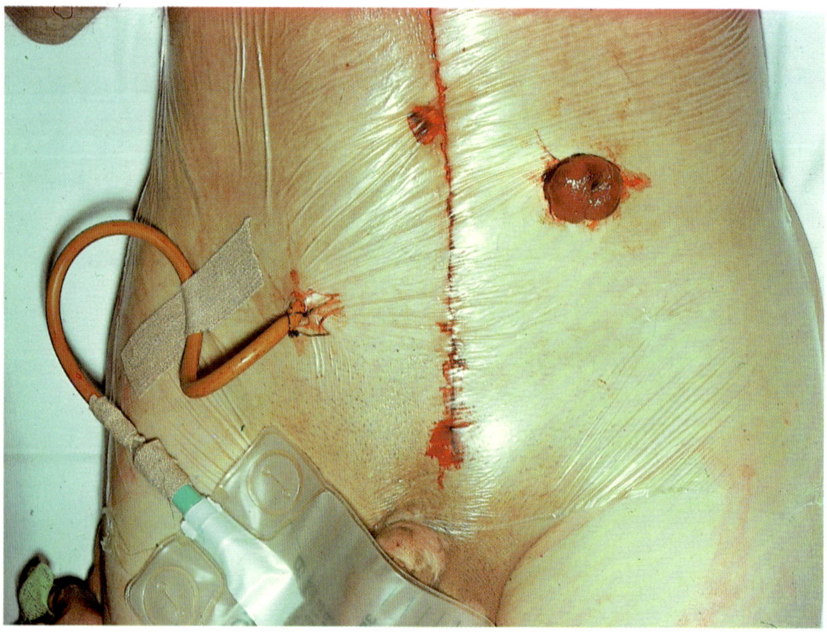

37 A left paramedian incision in a thin patient – as shown here – can interfere with the fitting of the adhesive plate of the appliance.

38

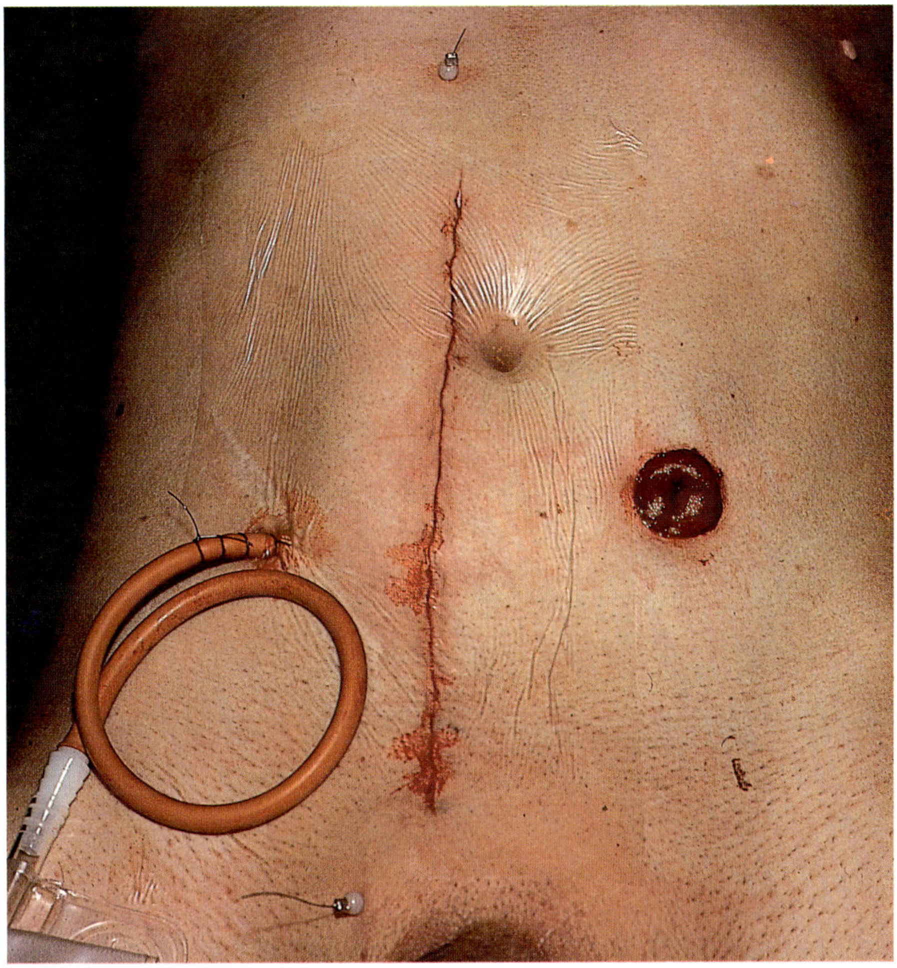

8 A right paramedian
ıcision is preferable in a thin
atient, though many surgeons
se a midline incision, which
aves both iliac fossae free of
cars.
Note the use of a subcuticular
itch held by beads (see
ection III) to obtain a neat
ar.)

39

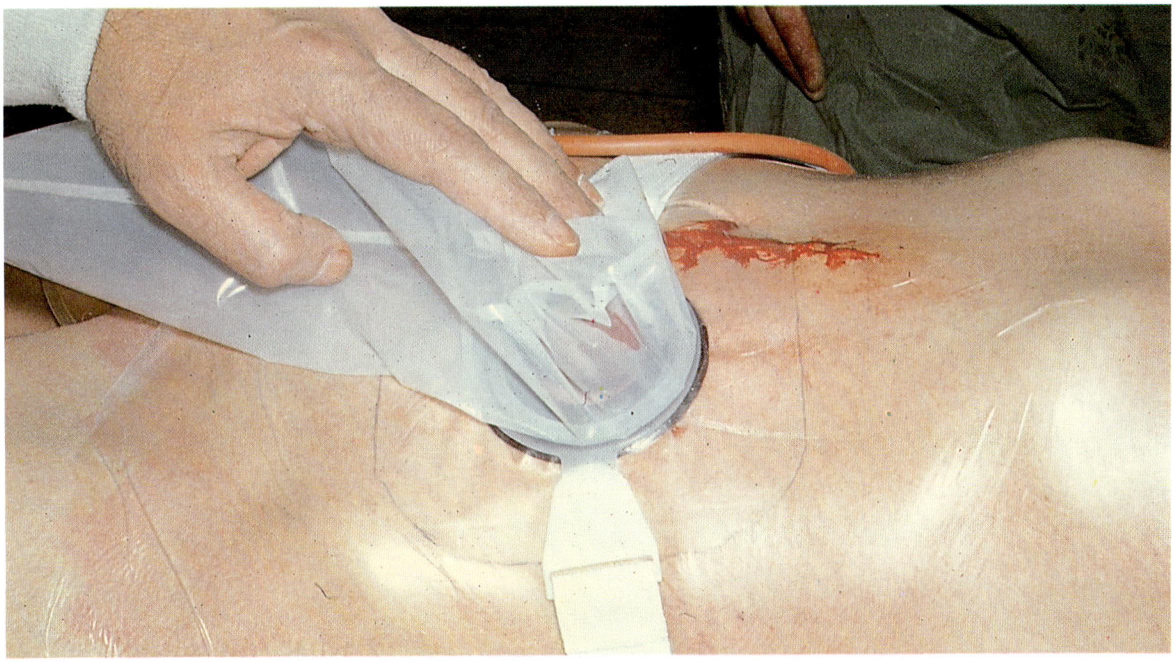

39 When correctly sited, the stoma lies midway between the waistline above and the hipline below. A light belt has been fitted to the appliance here to illustrate this point. The *wearing* of such a belt is not recommended.

CONSTRUCTING THE –STOMA
PART II: PREPARING THE SITE

Two techniques have been evolved:
A. The muscle splitting.
B. The trephine.

A. The muscle splitting technique

40
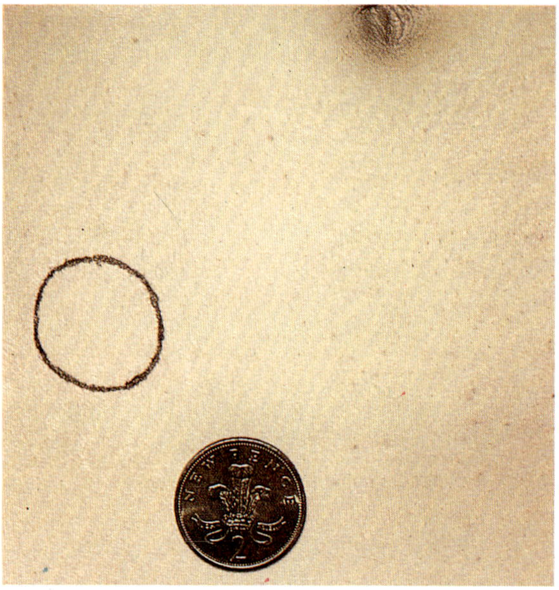

40 The hole is cut the size of a 2p piece (or quarter dollar, approx. 2.5 cm/1inch, see page 134) and the latter can be used to mark out accurately, with a skin pen, the site and size of the future stoma.

41
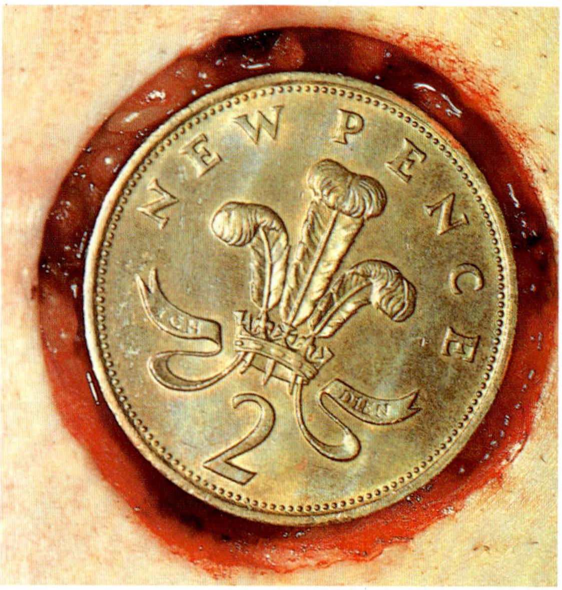

41 After skin excision, the edges retract centrifugally, so that the final diameter is slightly wider than the 2p piece.

42
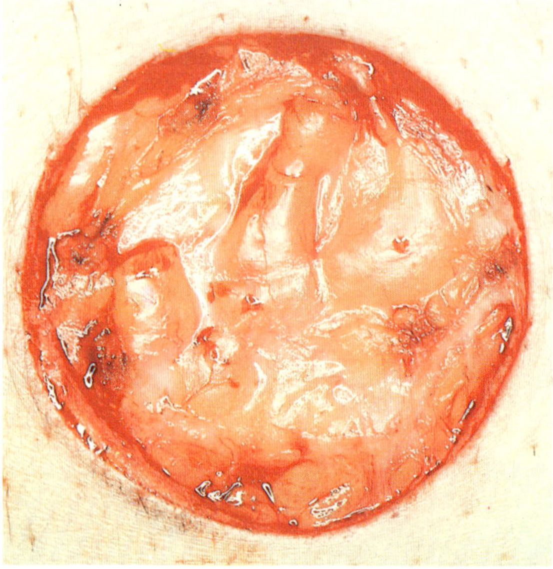

42 The 2.5 cm circle of skin is lifted off its underlying fat.

43
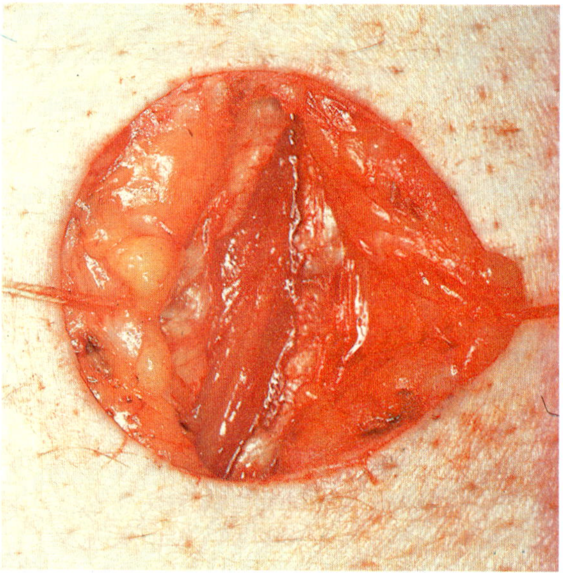

43 The fat is incised vertically down to the rectus sheath, which is in turn incised to expose the muscle.

44

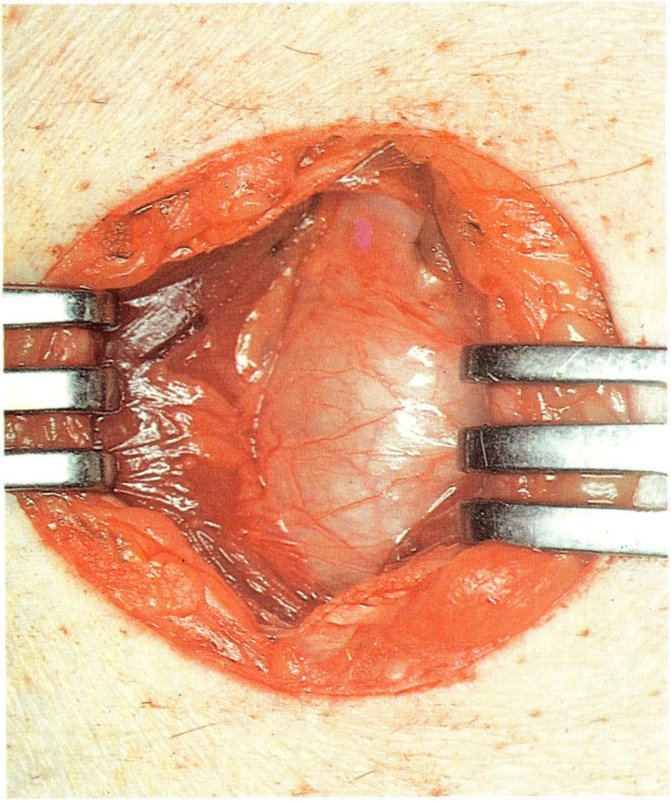

44 The muscle fibres are split and retracted to expose the posterior rectus sheath, avoiding separation of fibres from that sheath. Branches of the inferior epigastric artery may need to be divided and ligated.

45

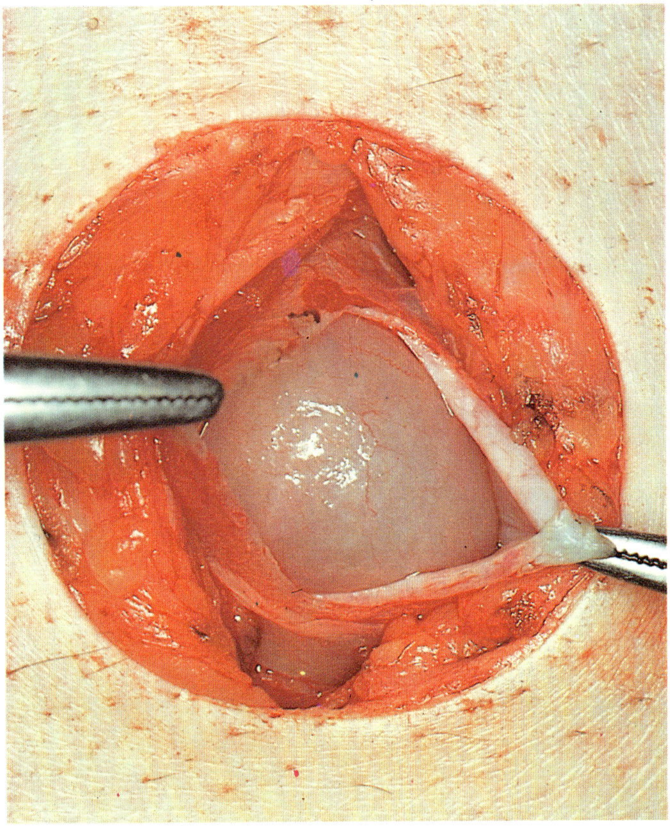

45 Finally, the posterior rectus sheath with its adherent underlying parietal peritoneum is divided in the same vertical line, which should be just long enough to accept the bowel. Too long an incision invites herniation.

B. The trephine technique

46
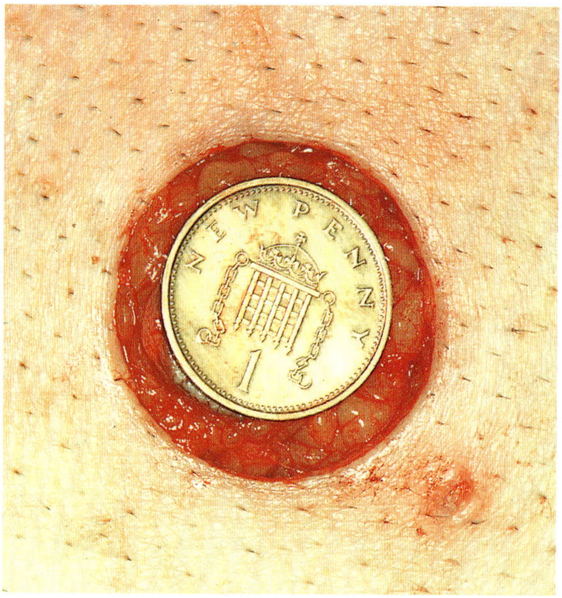

47
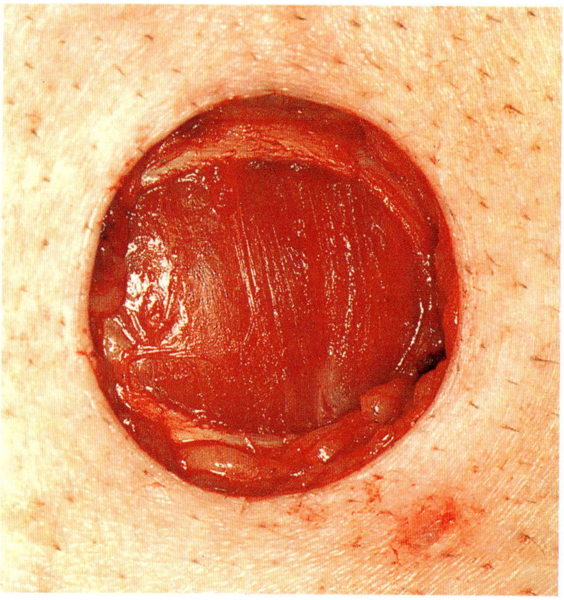

46 A smaller hole is advised to forestall herniation. A new penny piece provides a convenient size (2 cm (or a dime)) which, after skin retraction, produces a wider circle.

47 Subcutaneous fat and anterior rectus sheath are trephined out exposing the vertical fibres of the rectus muscle to the full diameter of the skin circle. (On occasions, the stoma may go through the external oblique.)

48
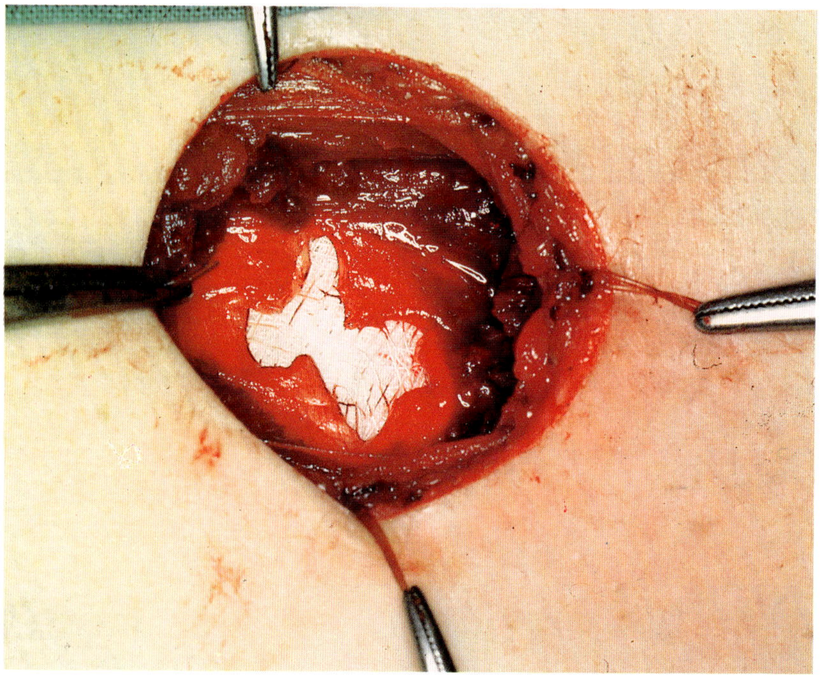

48 The rectus muscle is divided horizontally by diathermy to expose the posterior rectus sheath and peritoneum, which are in turn incised in a cruciform manner.

49

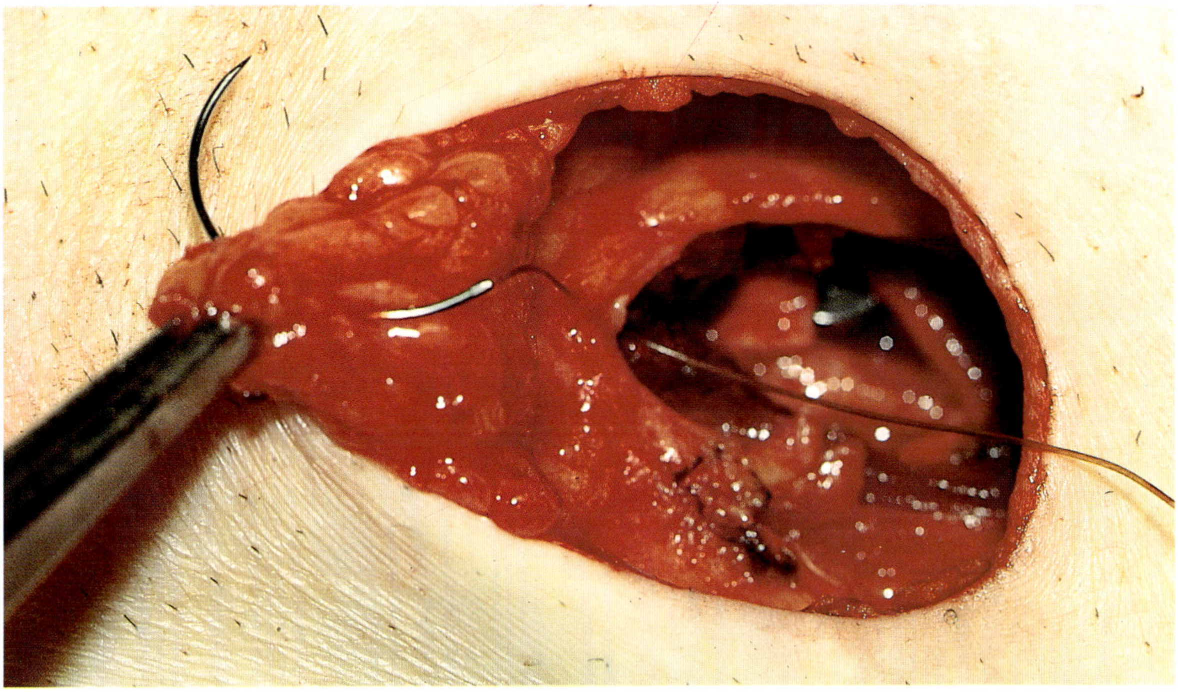

49 The edges of the subcutaneous space are sealed by sutures between the superficial fascia and the anterior rectus sheath. Four sutures are usually sufficient, and are a good precautionary measure against the formation of a para-stomal hernia.

50

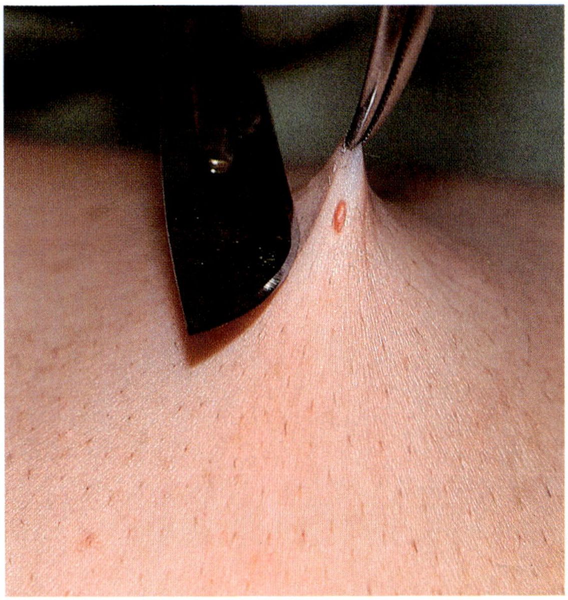

50 A popular and speedy method of excising a circle of skin is to tent it up at the chosen site, and with the scalpel held parallel to the abdominal wall to guillotine the cone of skin so formed.

51

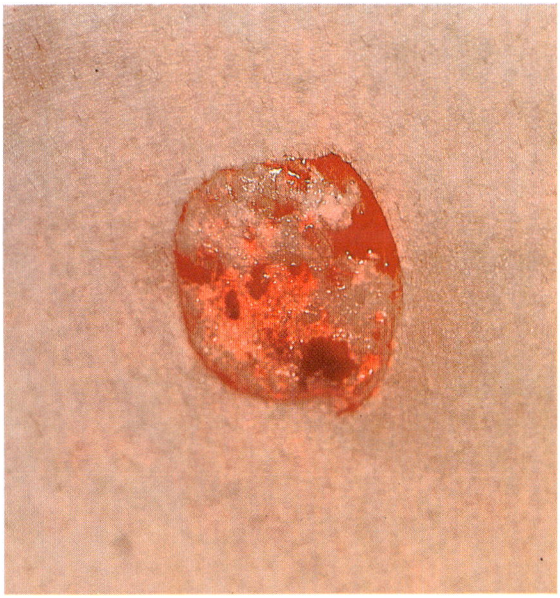

51 Its only drawback is that a circle of precise size and shape cannot always be obtained. The ragged contours often need correction if a perfect muco-cutaneous junction and a symmetrical stomal perimeter are the aims. It is however a favourite procedure in the hands of some experienced surgeons.

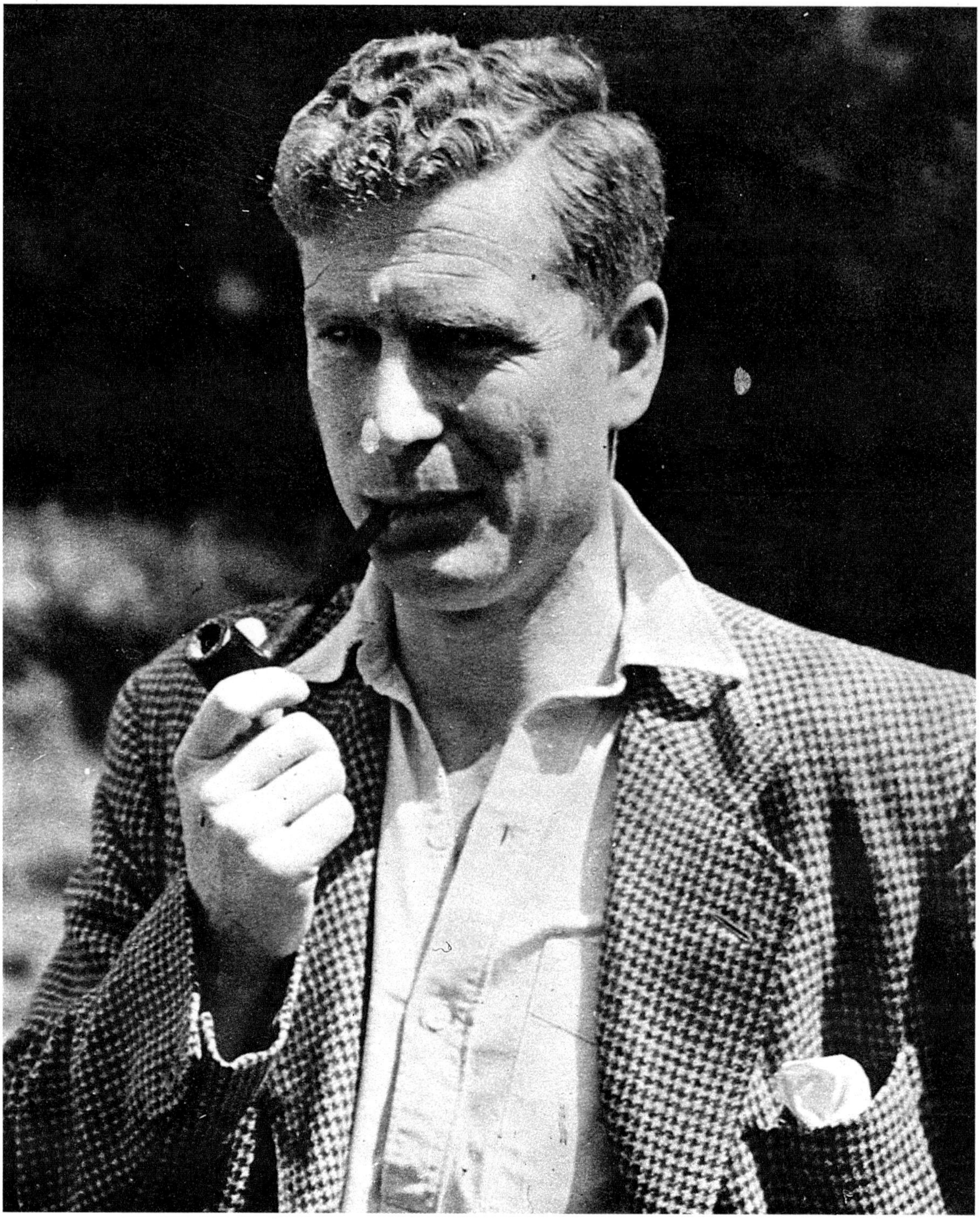

Professor Bryan Brooke

An informal photograph taken in 1952, the year he advocated eversion of the stomal spout and ushered in a new era in stomal surgery.

IV: CONSTRUCTING THE SPOUT

52
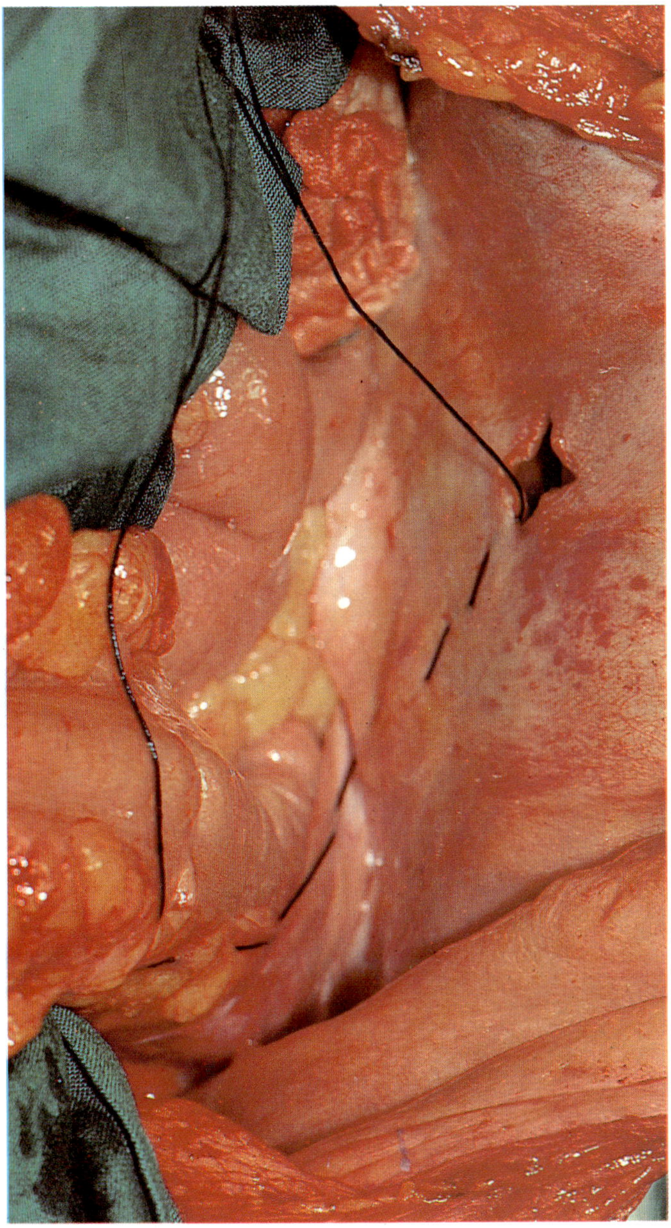

52 Fixation of the colon.

The prepared colonic loop is fixed to the antero-lateral wall of the iliac fossa by a purse-string of non-absorbable material, starting at the opening in the anterior parietes and coursing down the para-colic gutter to ascend the colon along its most appropriate taenia. Tying this suture not only fixes the colon to the anterior abdominal wall, but also obliterates the para-colic space. Note the clearly visible cruciate incision.

An alternative method is to prepare, between the posterior rectus sheath and the peritoneum, a tunnel through which the colonic loop is threaded to emerge at the site of the cruciate incision.

(In an ileostomy, the lateral space is closed by suturing the parietal peritoneum to the anterior wall peritoneum or, if of generous length, to the cut edge of the mesentery. Alternatively, it can be tunnelled under the parietal peritoneum. If the lateral space is wide, it need not be closed.)

53

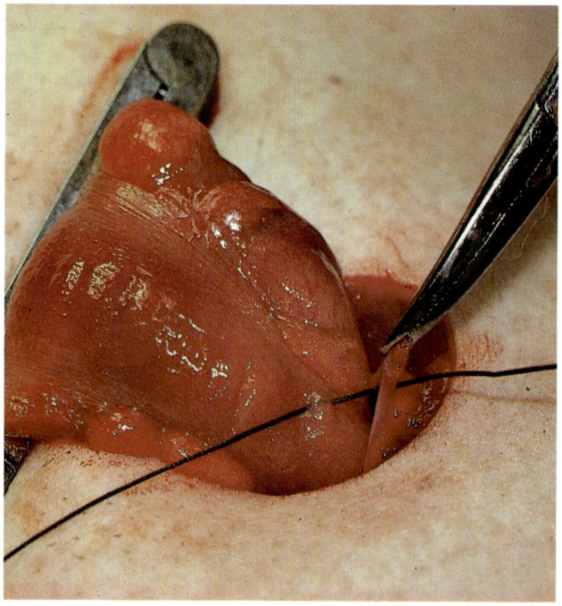

53 Further fixation to the abdominal wall is achieved by using the four triangles of tissue created by the cruciate incision. Unabsorbable material is used to attach each triangle to the colon by *no more* than its sero-muscular coat, to avoid the risk of fistula formation.

54

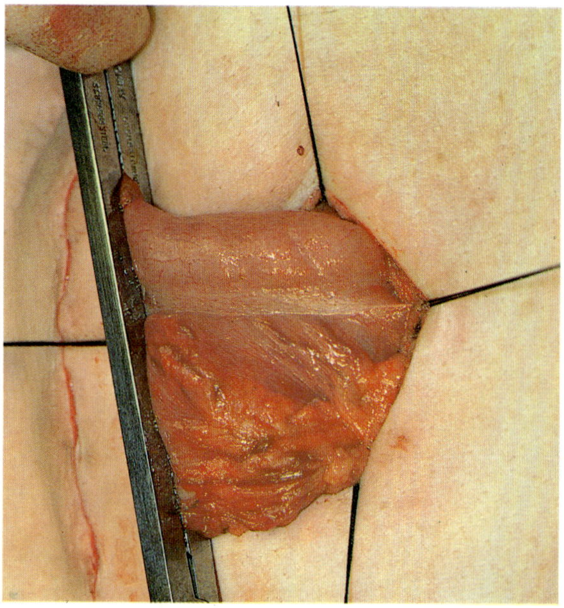

54 The four sutures in place, with the bowel fitting snugly within the trephined opening. They should now be cut close to their knots and the bowel allowed to sink in naturally. The spout is now ready for shortening if necessary, and then everted in readiness for the muco-cutaneous stitching.

Note that the abdominal wound has by now been closed and sealed.

55

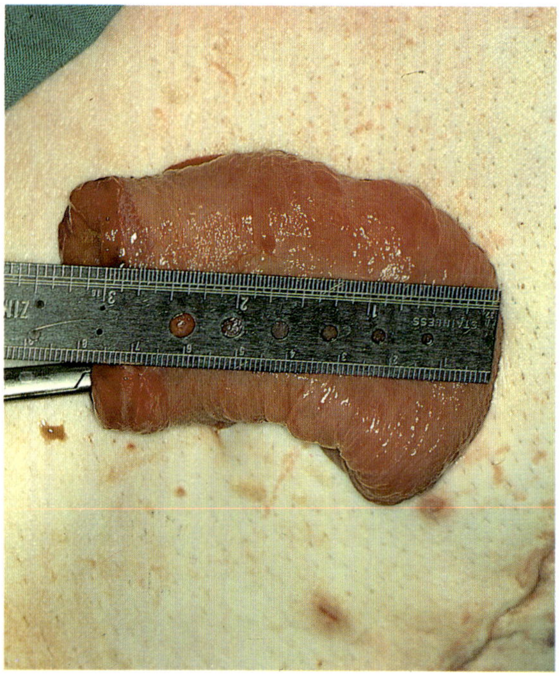

55 The length of bowel in an ileostomy should be 6–8 cm.

56

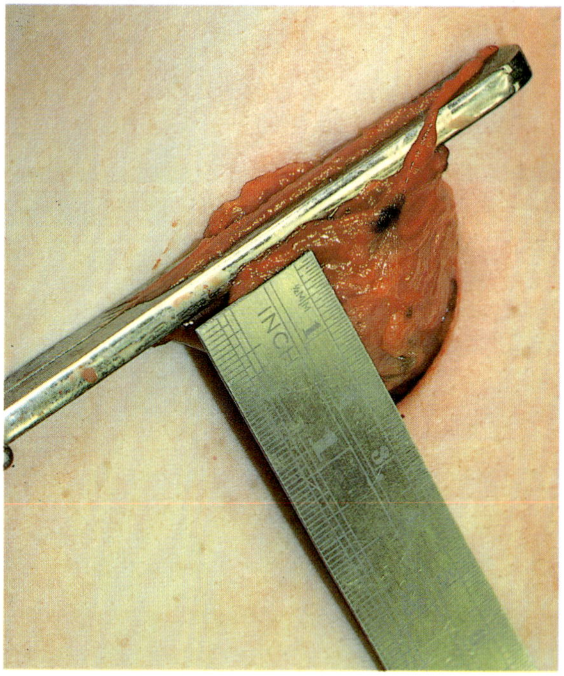

56 In a colostomy the corresponding length is 2–3 cm.

57

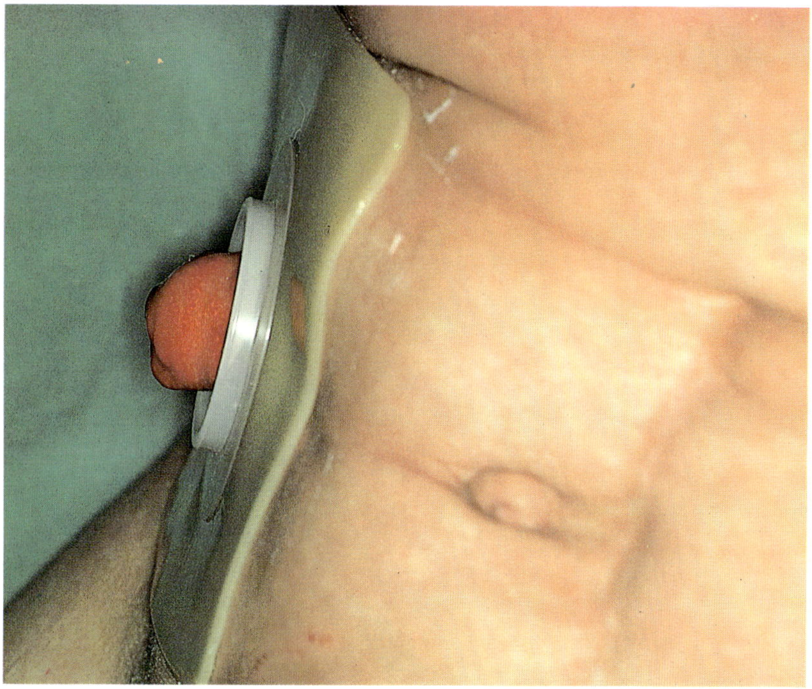

57 After eversion of 6–8 cm of ileum, a spout of some 3 cm remains. This should hang just over the appliance ring, allowing the more liquid ileostomy effluent to drip freely into the bag.

58

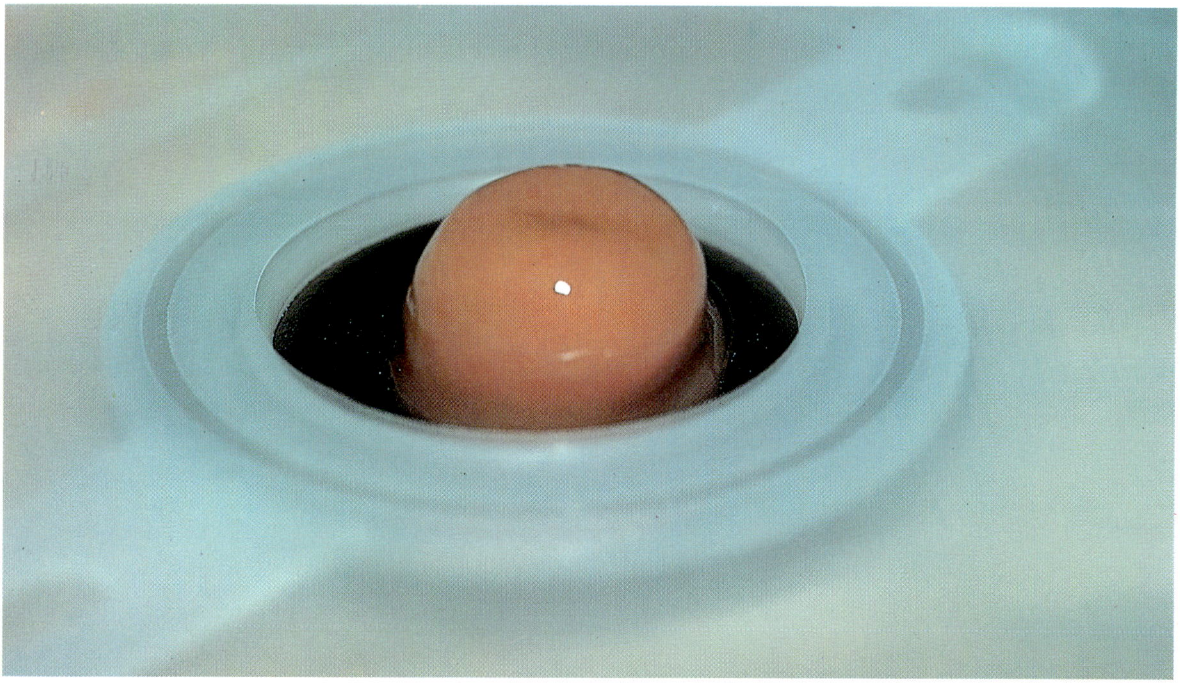

58 In the colon, eversion leaves a spout of 1 cm or just over, which projects slightly beyond the ring of the appliance.

V: THE MUCO-CUTANEOUS SUTURE

59

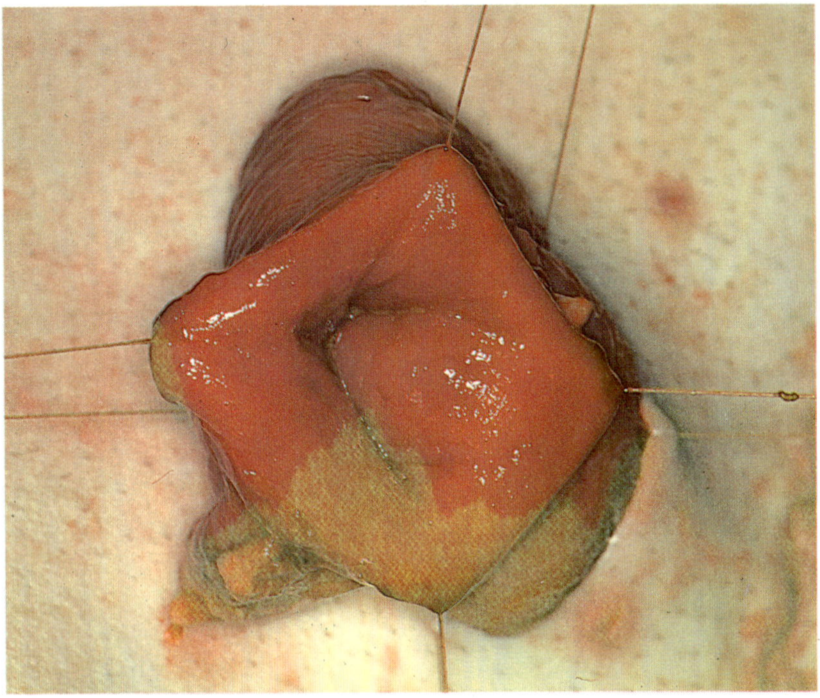

59 After removing the crushing clamp and securing exacting haemostasis of the bowel edge, the muco-cutaneous junction is sutured. Four stay sutures of 00 catgut are inserted through the full thickness of the skin to the full thickness of the bowel wall at the four cardinal points, the first step in the precise formation of the stoma.

60

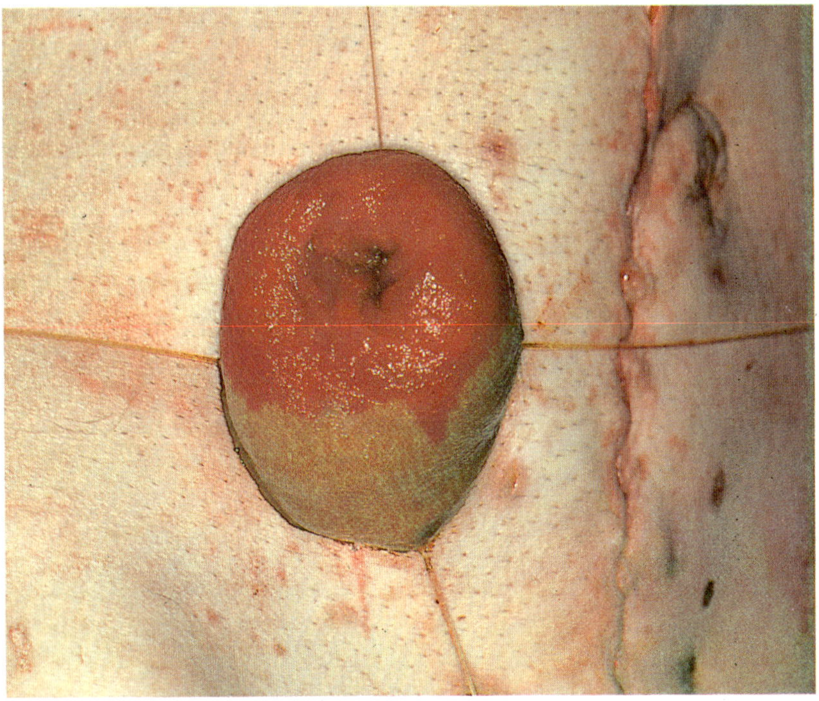

60 The four stay sutures are now tied, everting the bowel and fixing it evenly to the skin. When this suturing is completed the surrounding skin is firmly pressed upon, producing an even eversion of the whole bowel and creating – as seen here – a smooth stomal bud.

The latter is now ready for additional sutures between the four cardinal ones.

61

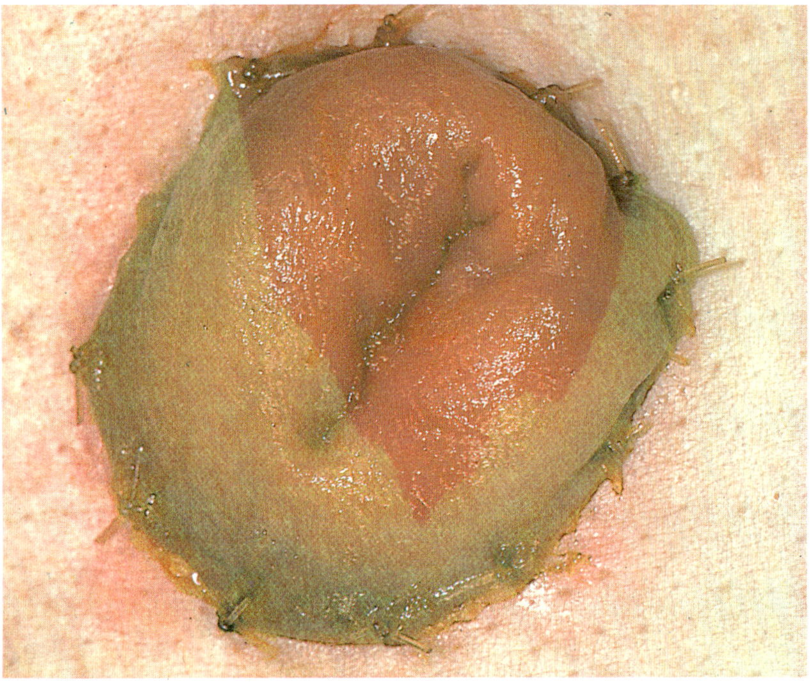

61 A colostomy with its muco-cutaneous suturing completed. Even and accurate stitching makes for early healing and a healthy muco-cutaneous junction. 00 or 000 catgut (see appendix) on a cutting needle is used by most surgeons.

62

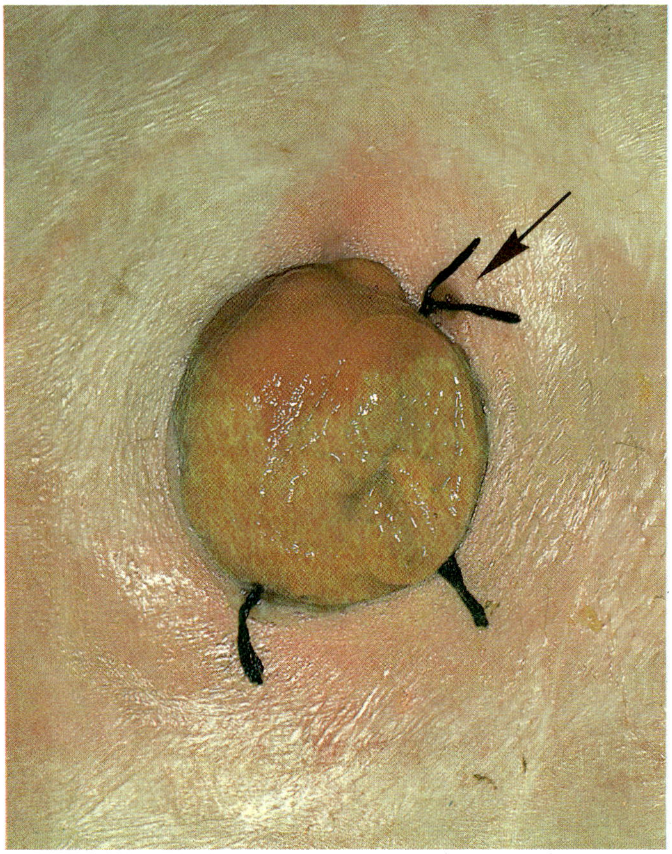

62 If non-absorbable sutures are used, they should be removed 7–10 days later. Here, silk sutures were 'forgotten' for 6 weeks!

63

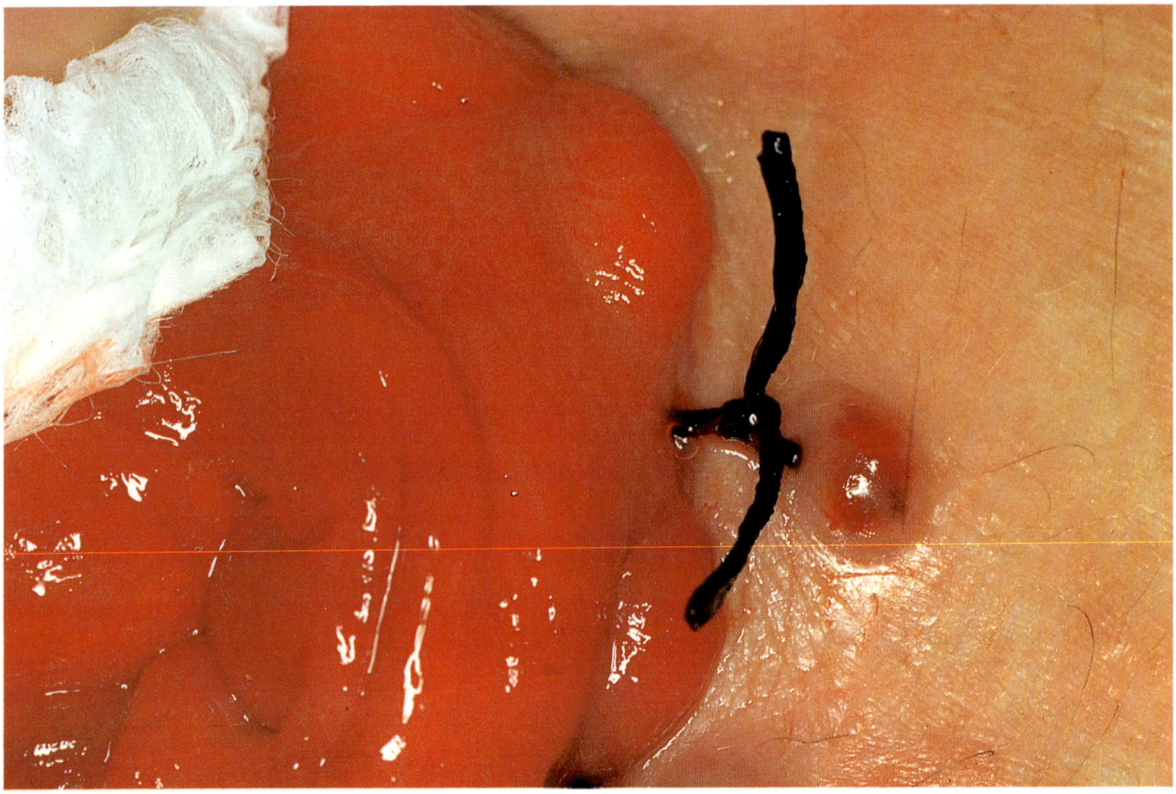

63 A close up of one of the sutures (arrowed in 62). A track has formed linking the mucocutaneous edge to the skin-exiting hole of the stitch. It was lined with colonic epithelium, and allowed faeces to leak under the appliance.

Its closure was speeded up by gentle curetting.

VI: CHOICE OF APPLIANCE

64

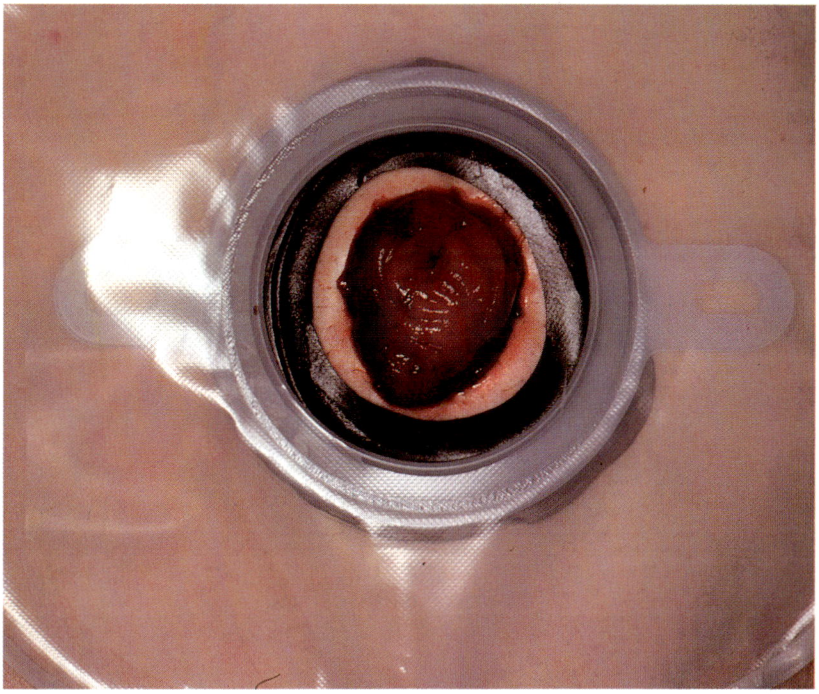

64 The initial appliance must be slightly bigger than the stoma. This allows for swelling of the stoma or the karaya gum washer.

65

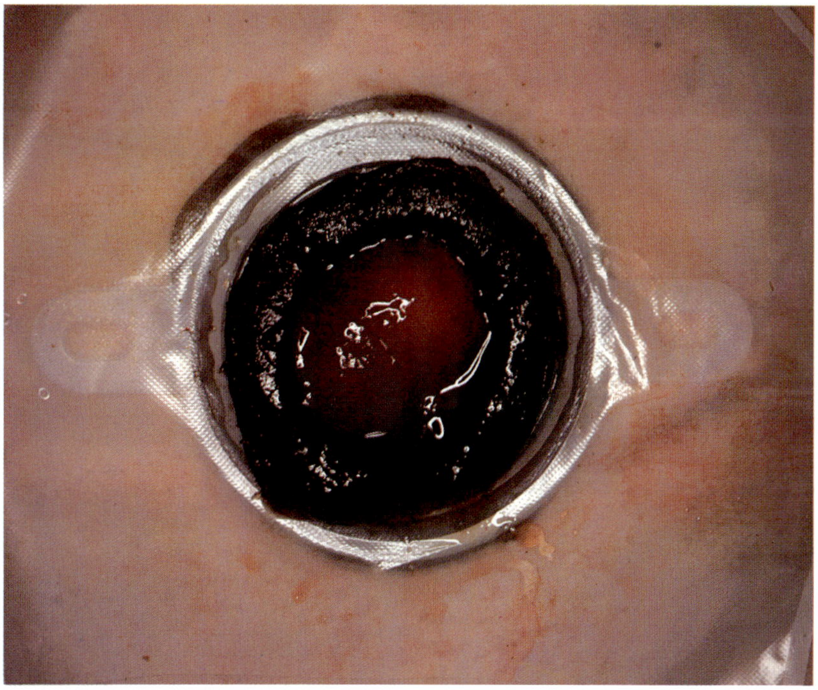

65 The same, 24 hours later. The swollen stoma is exuding mucus and serous fluid, leading to swelling of the karaya gum. A smaller appliance would have resulted in too tight a fit, and could cause mucosal damage or necrosis. Plum coloration and oedema are normal during the first few days, nonetheless the stoma should be inspected daily during this period, especially in the obese as they are more likely to have vascular impairment.

66

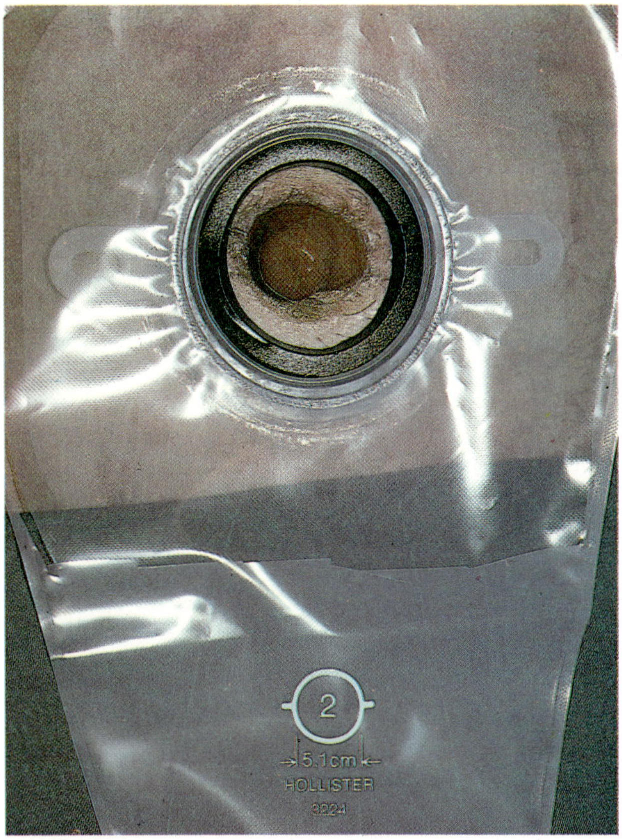

67

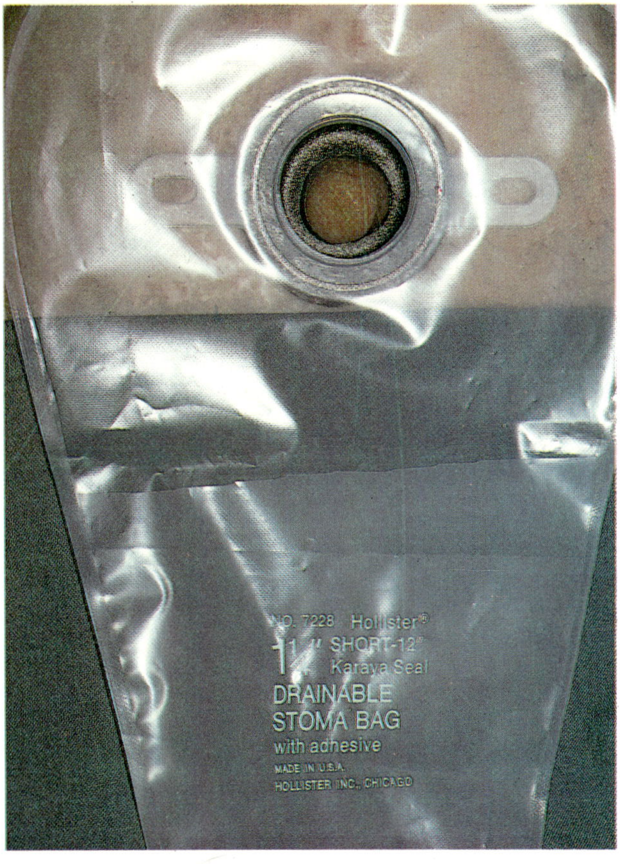

66 and **67** Four to six weeks later, the original 5 cm appliance will prove too large for the contracted stoma. It should be changed to the appropriate size, here 3 cm.

68

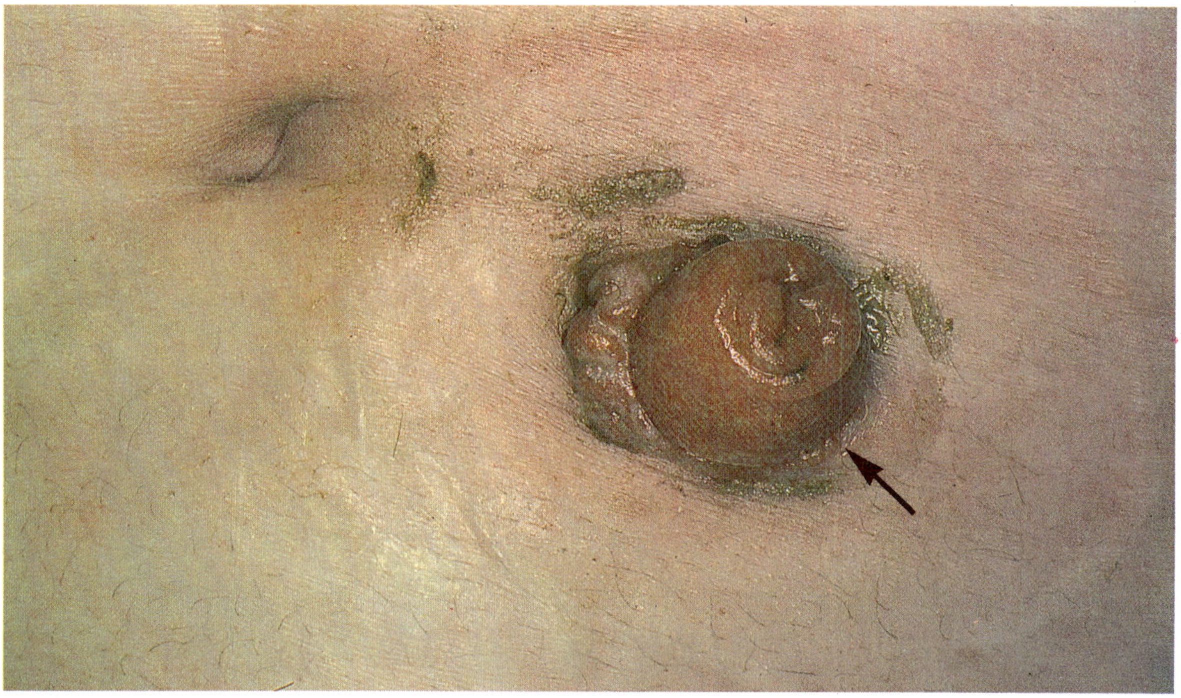

68 Too tight an appliance causes repeated trauma to the delicate muco-cutaneous junction. This leads to bleeding and the formation of small granulomas, claiming still more space within the flange. Contralateral pressure by the flange lip can then cause skin ulceration (arrowed).

69

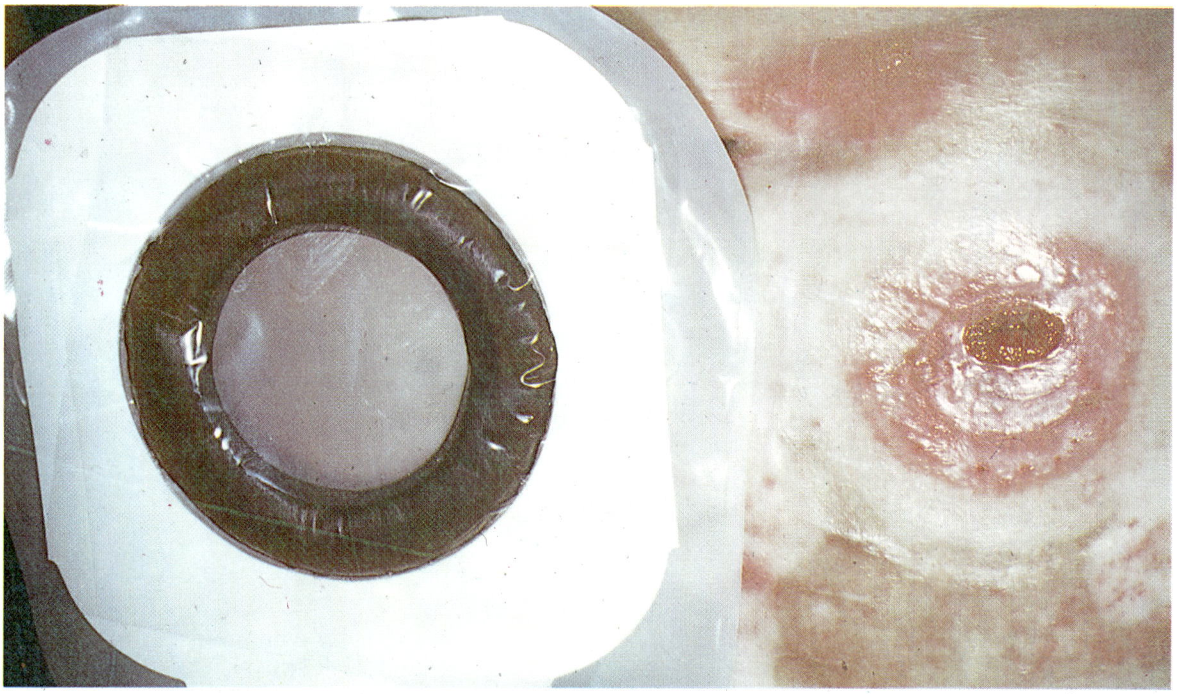

69 Too wide an appliance with damage to the skin within the flange by faecal dermatitis. Stenosis and stomal retraction have occurred. If in doubt about the right size of appliance use the measuring guide supplied by most manufacturers.

70

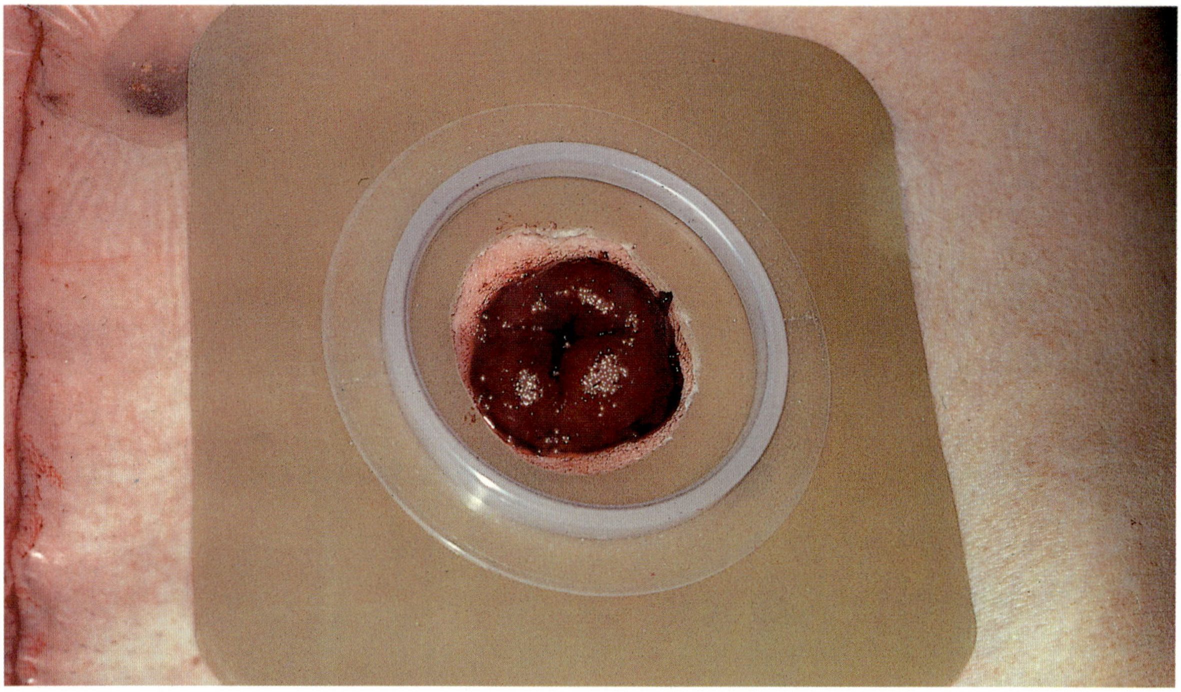

70 An alternative method is to use a 2-piece appliance with a plate (here of Stomahesive (see p. 122)) that can be holed as required, always starting with a slightly larger hole to allow swelling of the stoma.

Advantages: the hole can be progressively adjusted to fit the stoma; and the plate carries a clip-on disposable pouch, which need not be changed as long as it adheres satisfactorily.

Disadvantages: patients can cut the hole incorrectly and jaggedly, injuring the stoma if too small, or damaging the skin if too large.

71

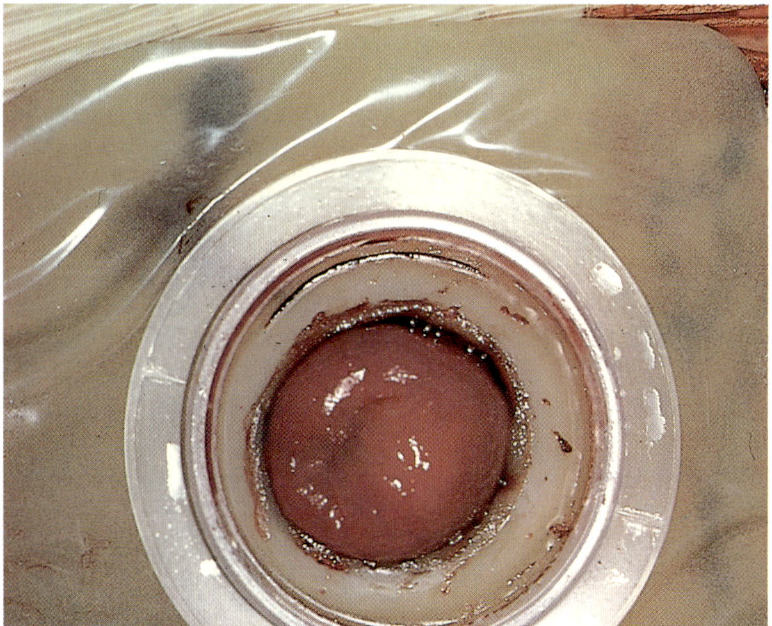

71 Swelling of the stoma and the Stomahesive (which is hydrophilic) fills in the gap between the former and the cut edges of the plate, making for a snug fit. (2nd post-operative day.)

VII: THE TRANSVERSE COLOSTOMY

The transverse colostomy

Transverse colostomies have certain features requiring special attention.

1. *Use*

It is primarily a temporary measure to defunction the distal colon, either decompressing it or diverting the faecal stream.

Decompression is either by a formal colostomy or by a 'blow-hole'.

2. *Construction*

(a) It must be fashioned at the site most suitable for wearing an appliance, usually midway between the subcostal border and the umbilicus.

(b) That site must be sufficiently close to the hepatic flexure to produce a short afferent loop, minimising the chances of prolapse.

(c) There should no tension on the afferent loop. Tension can cause retraction of the colostomy when the support rod is removed.

(d) The supporting rod or rubber tubing must be between the marginal artery and the colon, to avoid interference with the blood supply of the stoma.

(e) Supporting rods of various types have been produced, and can be fitted within an appliance. Alternatively, the rod can be tunnelled subcutaneously to hold the loop and is then clear of the appliance. Ox fibrin rods, which are subcutaneous and are absorbed within 3–4 weeks, give excellent results.

(f) Close the abdominal incision as snugly as possible round the loop. A loose closure invites herniation and prolapse.

(g) The colostomy should be opened on the operating table, attached by colocutaneous stitches and fitted with a bag immediately.

Loop colostomies simply held by a rod, opened 24–48 hours later, not capable of accepting an appliance, and with faeces spewing all over a distressed and depressed patient have been abandoned in units of excellence. Sadly enough, they are still practised by many but are to be condemned.

3. *Characteristics*

The effluent is semi-liquid and has a high enzyme content. Therefore good skin protection by a well-fitting appliance is essential.

Peristaltic movements are frequent and irregular. Such activity makes the colostomy somewhat incontinent and thus not easy to control – hence the necessity of an appliance from the start. It also makes the colostomy prone to prolapse. As the colostomy must start functioning immediately, an irrigation regimen is not suitable.

72

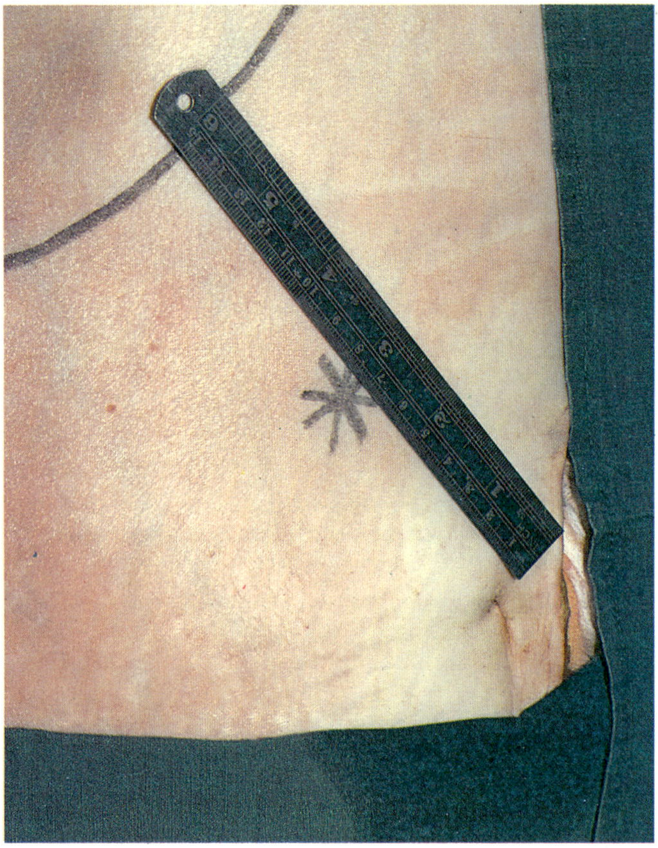

72 Select site pre-operatively if possible, by taking the midpoint of the line from the umbilicus to the nearest point on the costal margin.

73

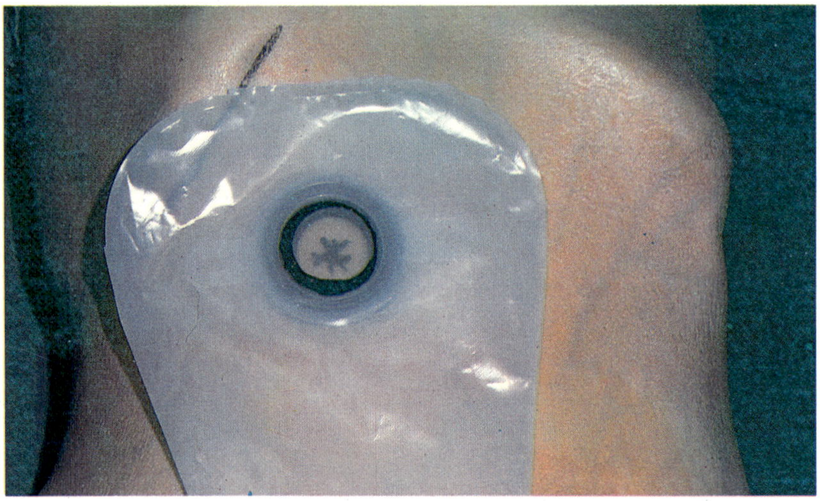

73 In an emergency situation the above siting will have to be relied upon. In elective cases, fix the appliance before operation to observe the suitability of the selected site.

74

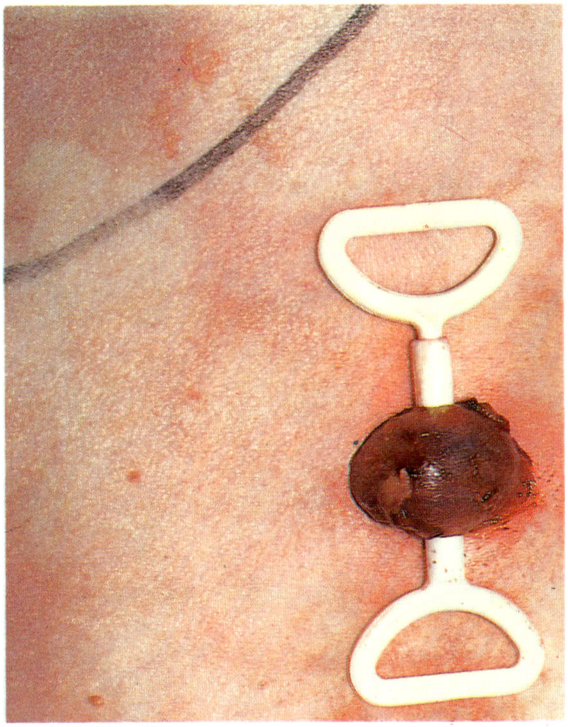

75

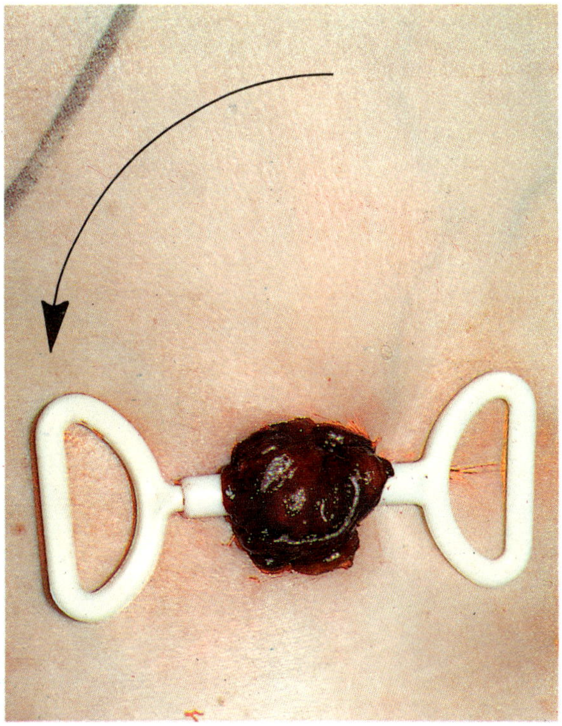

74 A trephine hole down to the anterior rectus sheath is the best incision; in a temporary colostomy use a 5 cm transverse skin incision. The colostomy loop, freed from omentum, is then brought out via a vertical incision through all remaining layers and kept exteriorised by a plastic rod (see appendix) inserted through the mesocolon between marginal artery and loop.

75 The rod is turned anti-clockwise through 90°, bringing the proximal loop inferiorly and the distal one superiorly. On opening the colon by a horizontal incision, the barrels will lie in a vertical plane with the distal loop lying above the active one – a manoeuvre that improves the defunctioning of the former and is said to minimise herniation and prolapse.

76

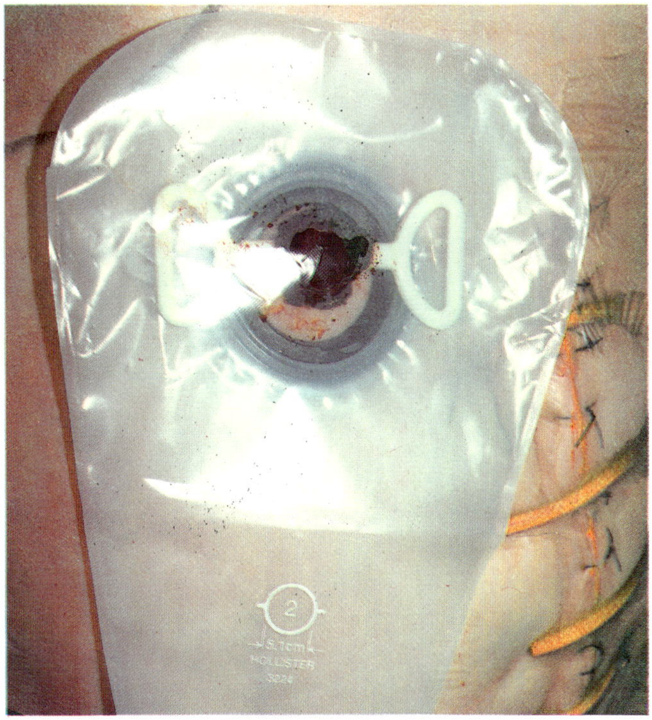

76 Muco-cutaneous sutures of catgut are inserted as usual, saddling the colostomy over the rod. Use appliance with a large hole to accommodate the rod that lies across its ring.

77

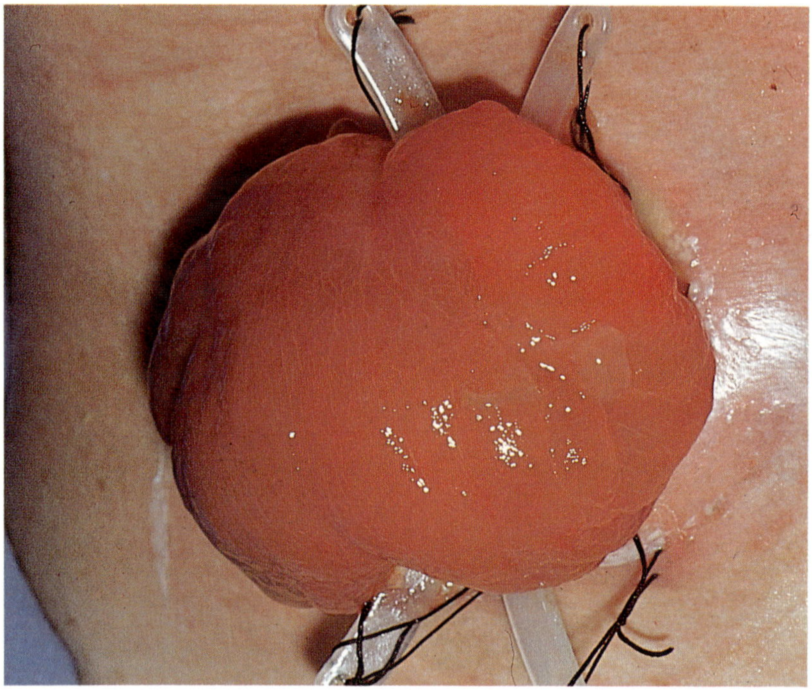

77 Another frequently used colostomy support is the plastic cross. It is fixed by skin sutures through holes as shown. Too tight an abdominal aperture, or too taut a loop can lead to early oedema of the stoma as seen here. This usually disappears on removing the support.

78

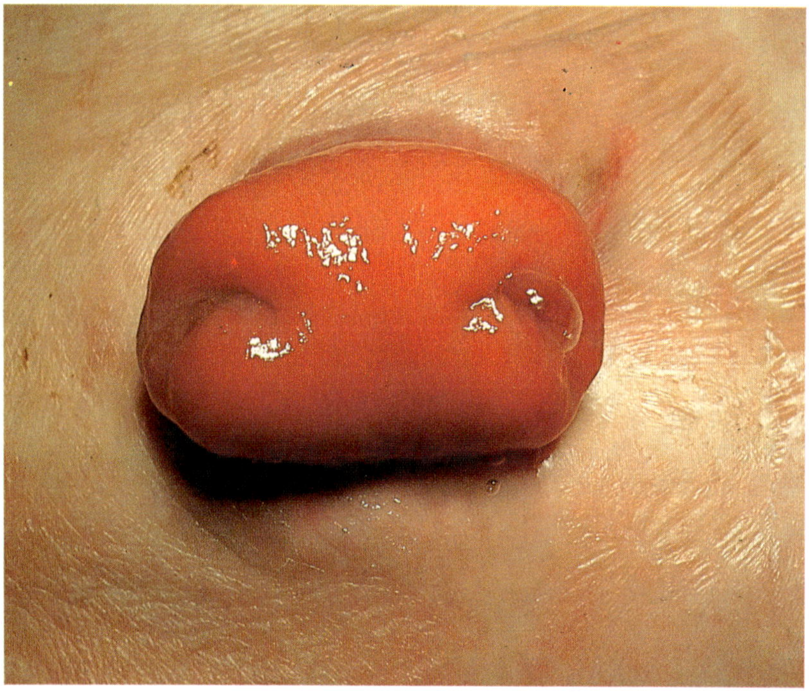

78 The colostomy a few weeks later with its typical double barrel appearance.

79

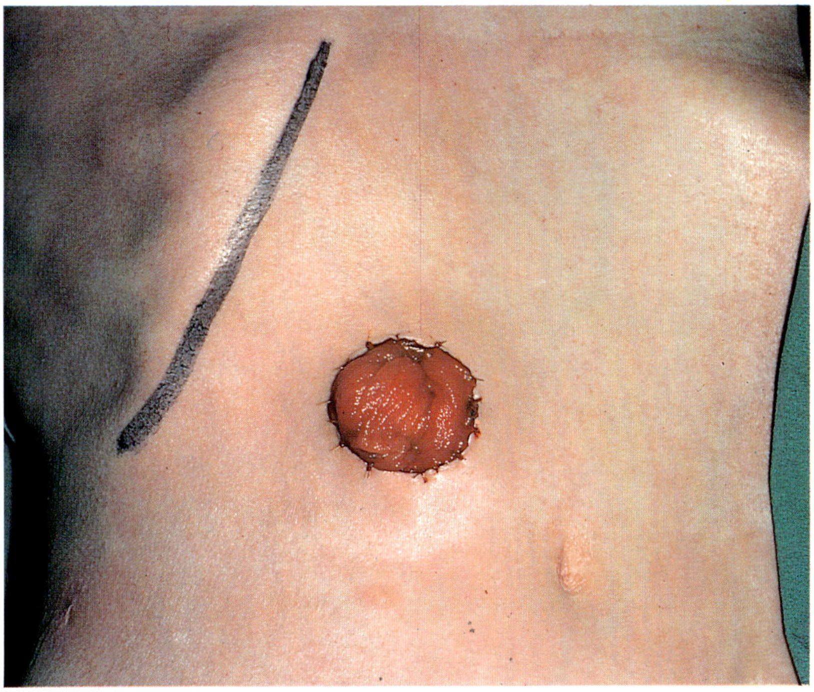

79 The best colostomy support is that made of ox fibrin (Biethium; see appendix). It is buried at operation, thus allowing a neat muco-cutaneous suturing of the colostomy, shown here with its barrels again in a vertical plane.

80

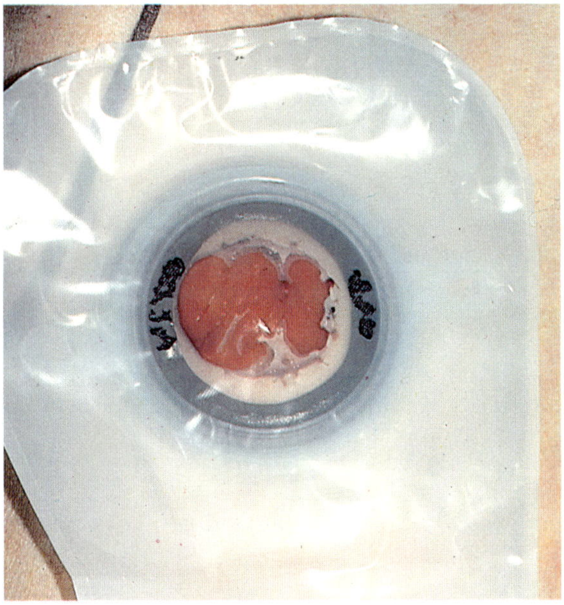

80 A standard appliance is fitted and managed in a way no different from that used in a straightforward left iliac colostomy.

81

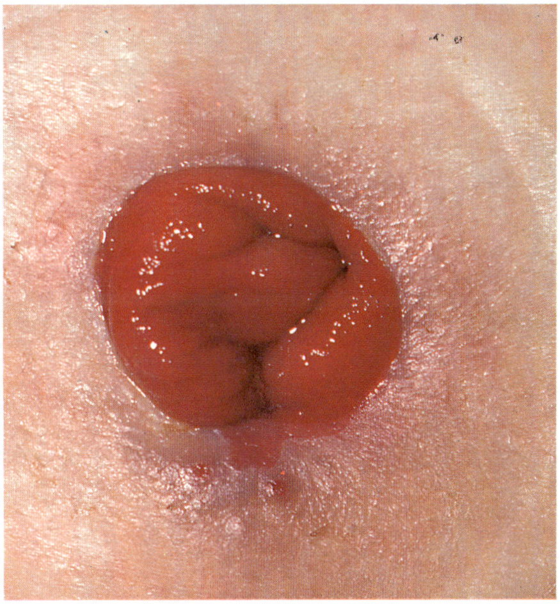

81 The 'mature' colostomy a few months later – free of herniation or of prolapse. This method of constructing a double barrel defunctioning colostomy gives very gratifying results.

VIII: THE ILEOSTOMY EFFLUENT

82
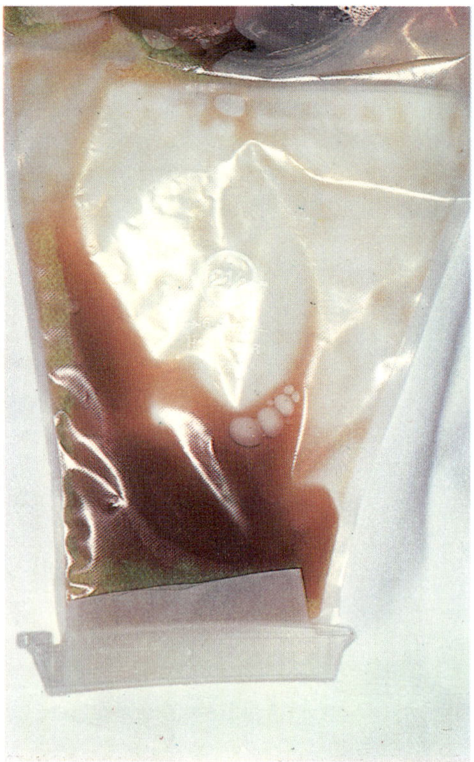

83
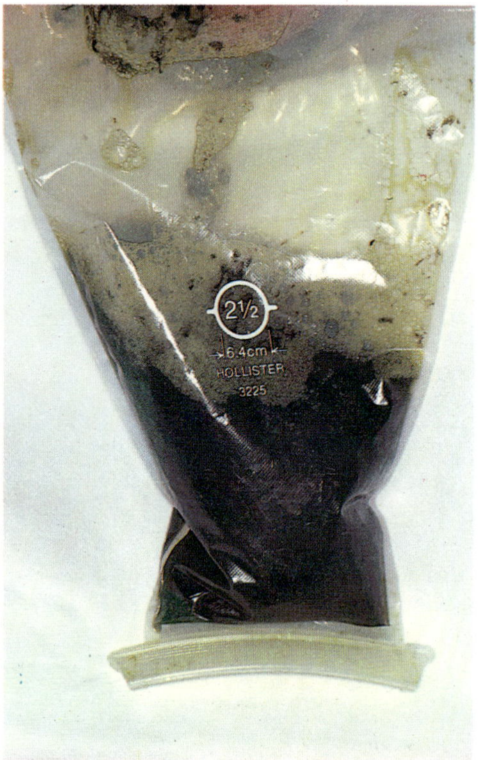

84
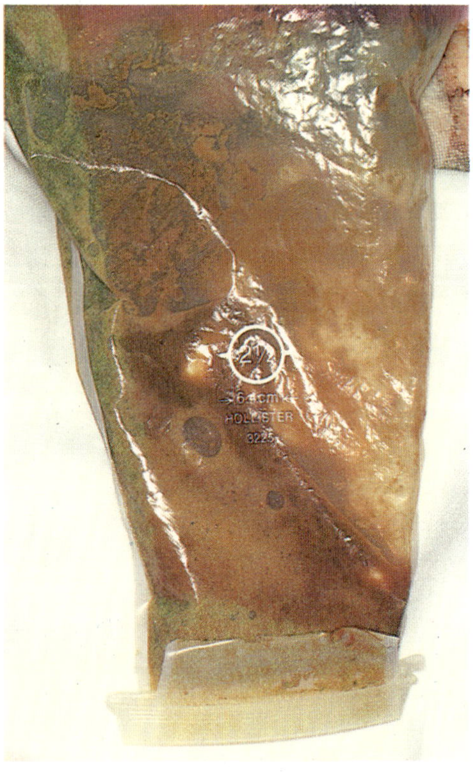

82 Blood stained serous fluid accumulates in the bag in the first 24–48 hours and is a normal occurrence.

83 The first effluent, once peristalsis returns, is commonly thin and bile stained, reflecting the starved condition of the small bowel and the still impaired enterohepatic circulation.

84 After feeding, the effluent thickens, as bile and fluids are reabsorbed by the gut. Its volume diminishes markedly and it becomes olive-brown.

IX: THE PERINEAL WOUND

The perineal wound

There are several good methods of dealing with the perineal wound, depending on the nature of the lesion, and the sex of the patient:

(a) **Primary closure** with drainage above or below is usually performed in the male.

(b) Primary perineal closure with **posterior vaginal excision**, without its reconstruction. This is performed with malignancy, but not for inflammatory bowel disease.

(c) **Partial perineal closure**, the 'semi-closed' method, with perineal drainage.

(d) **Anal preservation.** This may be partial, using an inter-sphincteric dissection, or total, using a pull-through method.

(e) Use of a **pedicled omental graft** to fill the pelvic space and refashion the perineum.

Packing is not recommended as a routine procedure, but may be necessary to control haemorrhage.

Primary closure

Primary closure is the ideal reconstruction to be aimed at in men, regardless of the lesion, and in women with inflammatory bowel disease.

After excision, the wound is irrigated with chlorhexidine or with sodium hypochlorite and closed as completely from below as possible. Interrupted silk sutures can be used, but subcuticular nylon seems more comfortable. Similarly, drainage from above allows the patient greater mobility with less discomfort, though perineal drainage is still very popular with surgeons. Whichever method is used, suction should be applied for 4–5 days, or until the daily discharge falls below 15 ml.

Partial perineal closure

If total closure is not possible, the middle part of the wound is left open and a drain – usually corrugated – stitched in.

Primary perineal closure with posterior vaginal excision

In women, because local recurrence of malignancies are usually in the recto-vaginal septum, it is wise to excise the posterior vaginal wall. The fourchette is reconstructed and the skin closed, but the vaginal wound is not sewn up, and is allowed to granulate. This will preserve the normal size of the vagina. The drain is then placed through the vaginal wound.

In inflammatory bowel disease in women, the perineum is treated as in the male closed method, the posterior vaginal wall being preserved and a primary complete closure effected.

When fistulae are present – as in Crohn's disease – they are best removed *en bloc* with the anus. But when tracks are long, they should be laid upon and curetted. Sometimes curetting alone is sufficient. Primary closure is not always possible in these cases.

Anal conservation – only acceptable in selected cases of inflammatory bowel disease – preserves the anatomy of the vagina and perineum in young women and may reduce sexual dysfunction in men. An intersphincteric dissection can be carried out, or the rectal stump can be invaginated within itself, pulled through and divided at the ano-rectal verge, which is then closed completely.

Primary closure breaks down in 25–30% of all cases, more so in inflammatory bowel disease. However, if omentum is brought down into the pelvis and used as a graft, filling the pelvic space and cushioning the perineum, very gratifying results are obtained, more so when wide skin excision has to be undertaken as in Crohn's disease.

Accidental transgression of the rectal wall with escape of its intra-luminal contents increases several-fold the rate of local recurrence. Wash-out with mercuric perchloride (1:500) may diminish the chances of malignant cell seeding, but may cause renal damage.

Sutures are best left for at least ten days, but should not stop the patient from having daily baths.

85

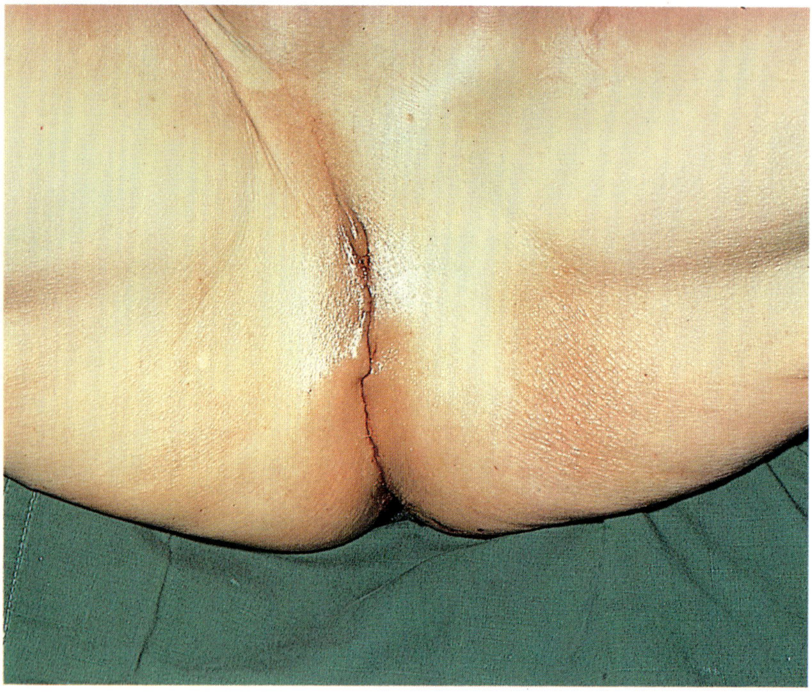

85 Abdomino-perineal excision in the male. Complete the primary closure, using suprapubic drainage. (See **37**.) A polyglycolic acid subcuticular stitch has been used here.

86

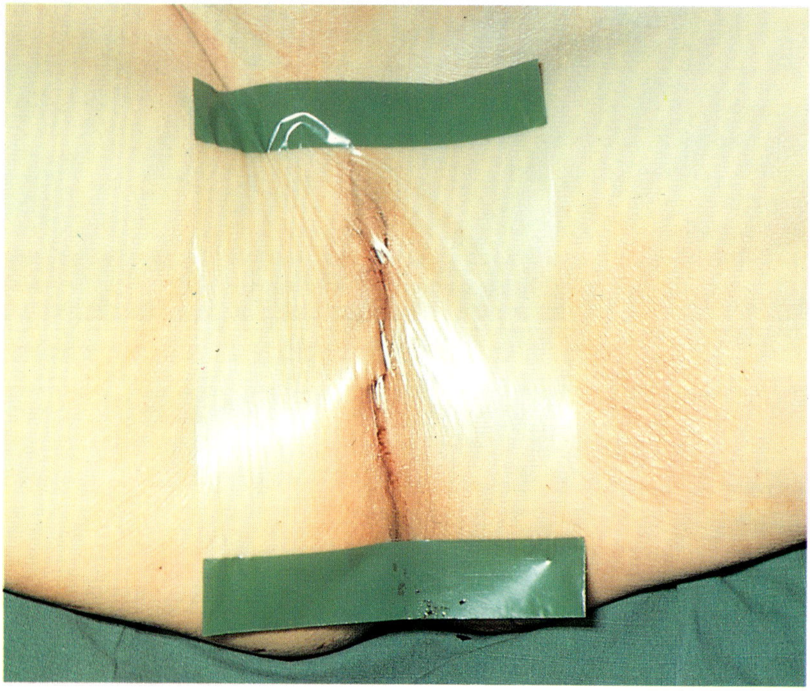

86 A semi-permeable drape is used as a dressing to seal off the wound. It is comfortable, reduces perineal wound nursing to a minimum, and keeps the wound dry during the daily baths in the early post-operative days.

87

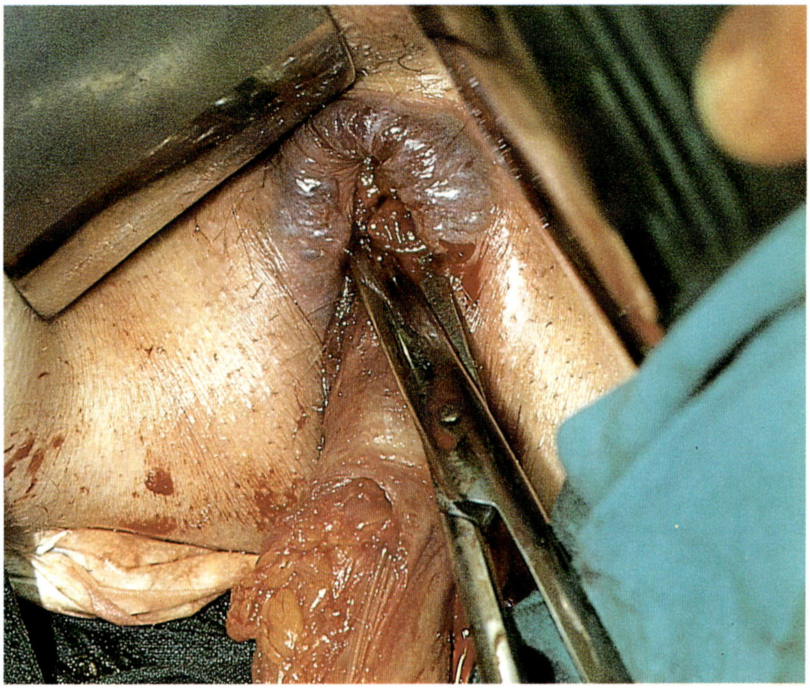

87 Anal preservation. Young male with ulcerative colitis.

The rectum has been exteriorised by a pull-through manoeuvre and is being divided on the anal side of the ano-rectal junction. The anus is then completely closed using interrupted catgut sutures. The omentum was too thin and too short to be used as a graft here.

88

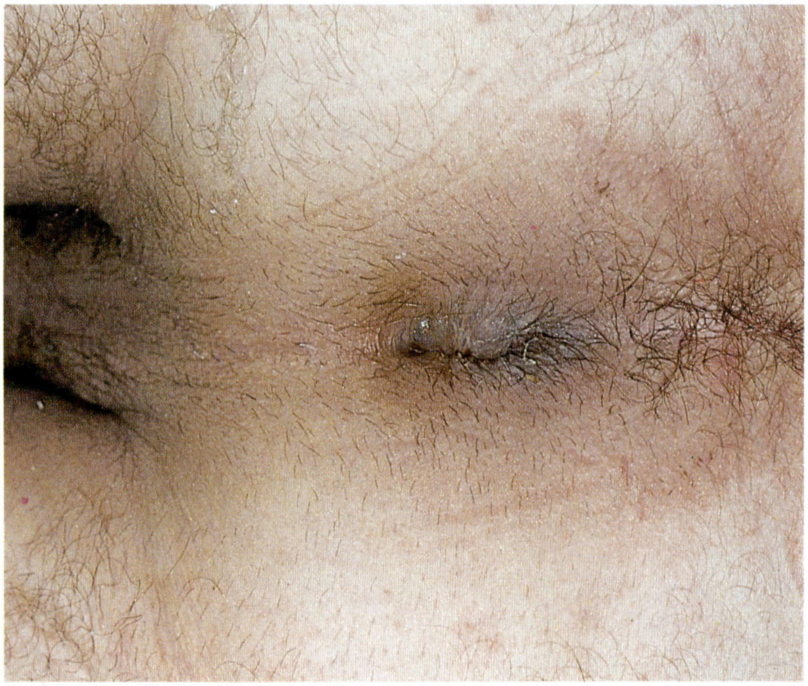

88 The same patient four weeks after surgery. The wound healed by first intention, and hardly needed any nursing care in the post-operative week. The patient is lying in the right lateral position.

89

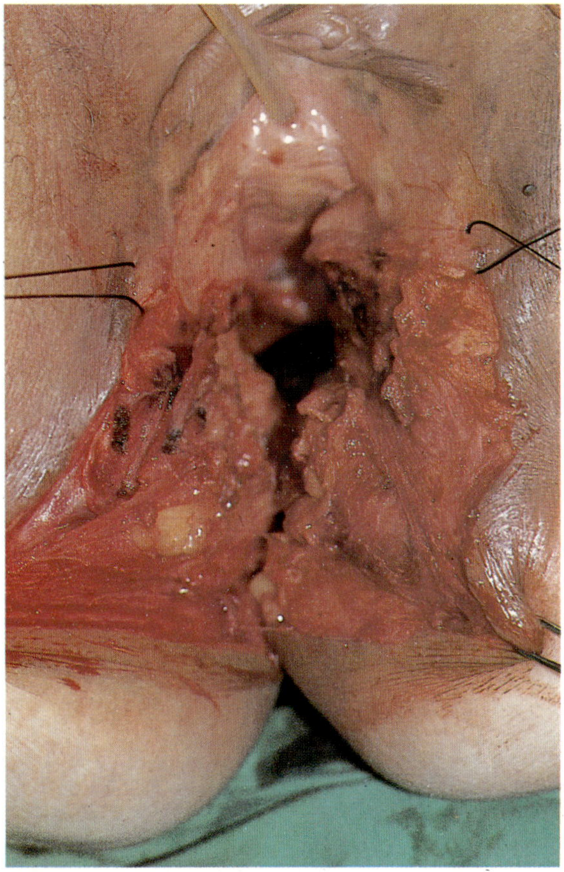

89 The semi-closed method. An abdominoperineal excision of a rectal carcinoma in a sixty year old woman. The posterior wall of the vagina has been removed with the rectum. The two silk stitches are at the lower limits of the introitus, and are useful landmarks in the perineal reconstruction.

90

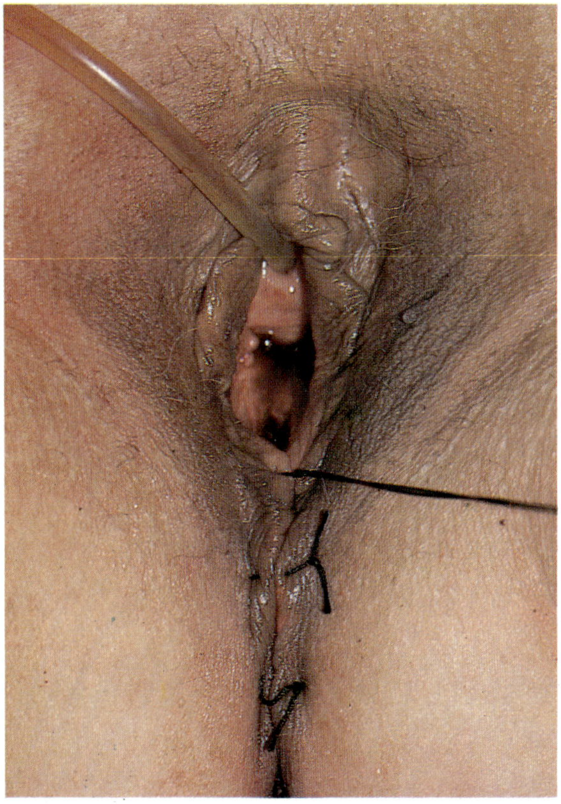

90 Same patient as above. The deeper layers have been closed with catgut. A new fourchette has been reconstructed, approximating the edges of the posterior vaginal wall only at the introitus; while the deeper portion is left open. The rest of the perineal wound has been closed with interrupted silk sutures.

91

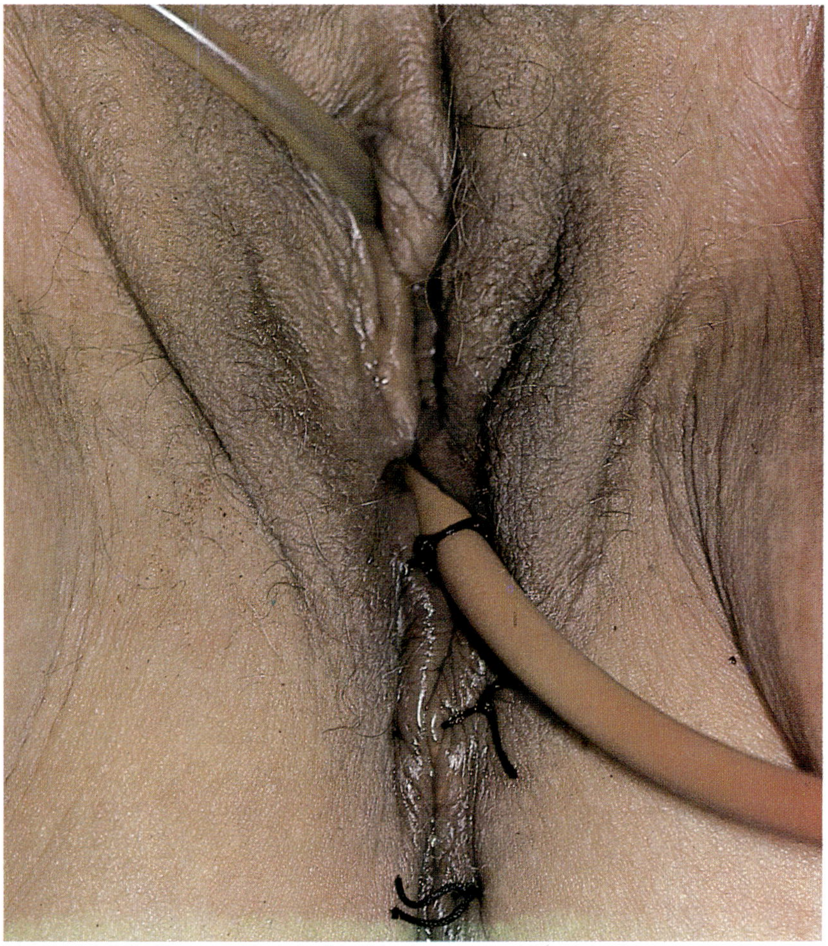

91 A tube drain is inserted via the open vaginal wound into the deeper perineal space created by the excision. The stitch at the fourchette conveniently anchors it in that position. The drain is removed once the daily discharge falls below 15 ml.

92

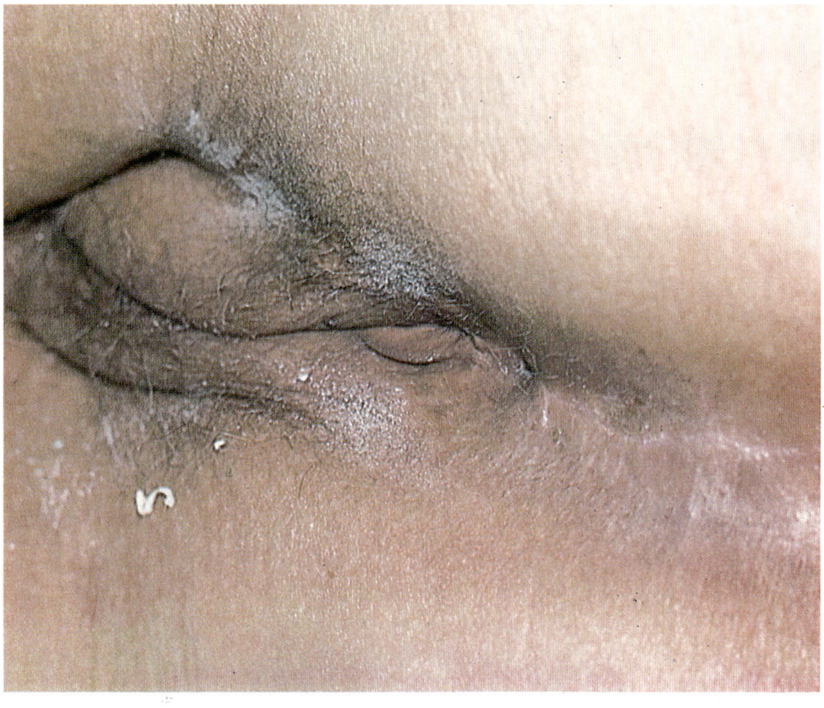

92 The same wound four weeks later (the patient lying in the right lateral position). The patient had been discharged home on the 12th post-operative day; the sutures were removed on the 10th day.

At the time of going home all discharge had stopped. The posterior vaginal wound had united at several points with islands of granulating tissue in between.

At four weeks the posterior vaginal wall had totally re-epithialised. There was no bladder dysfunction.

93

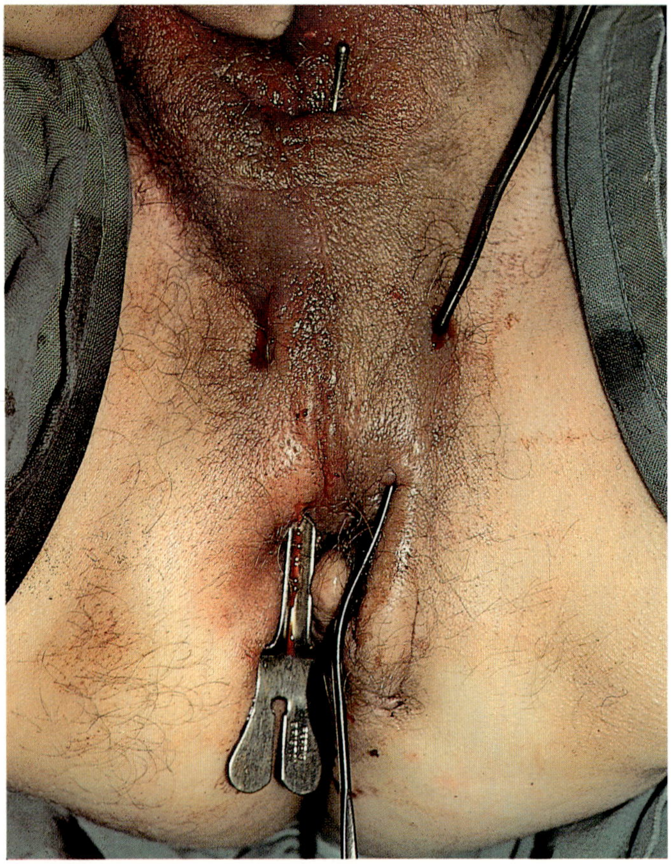

93 Male with Crohn's disease and perineal fistulae.

The one on the left was excised with the anus. The ano-scrotal one was partly excised and partly curetted. An omental graft was used to fill the pelvic cavity, and primary wound closure was successfully undertaken.

94

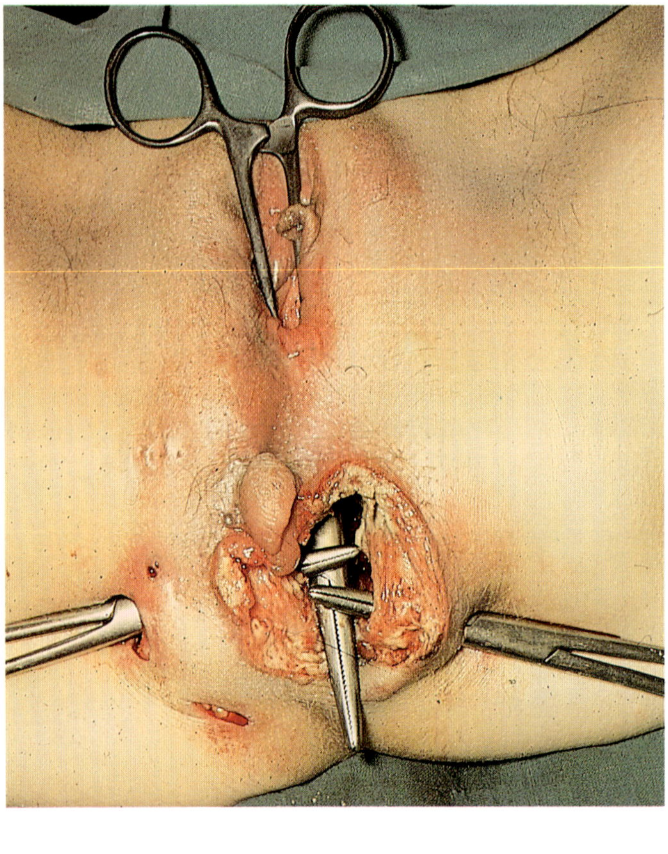

94 Severe Crohn's disease in a young woman. The anus has been almost totally destroyed; and a wide ano-vaginal fistula required excision of the outer part of the posterior vaginal wall.

The semi-closed method was used here, with omentum packing the pelvic cavity. It supported the deep aspect of the posterior vaginal wall, and offered a well vascularised bed for granulation tissue to bridge the lost vaginal wall behind the fourchette.

95

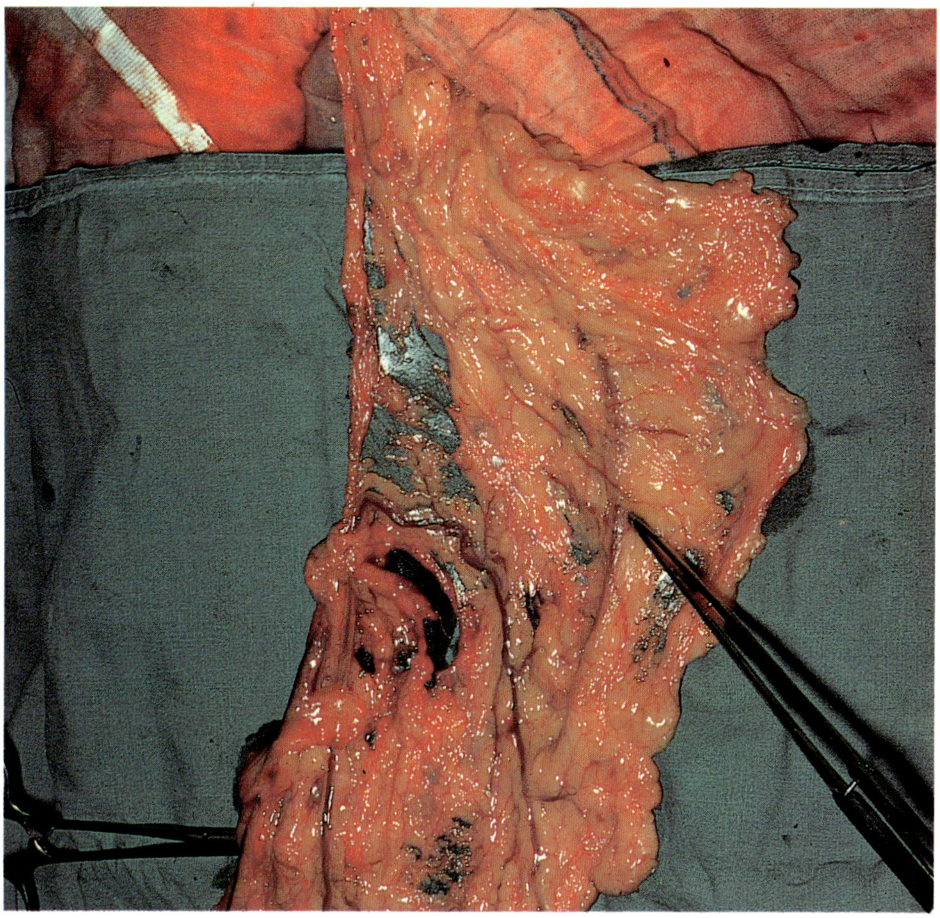

95 The omental graft. The mobilised omentum before it is brought down to the perineum. The pedicle is based on tissue vascularised by the left gastro-epiploic vessels (indicated by the dissecting forceps). Every effort is made to preserve all the vascular branches of that artery.

96

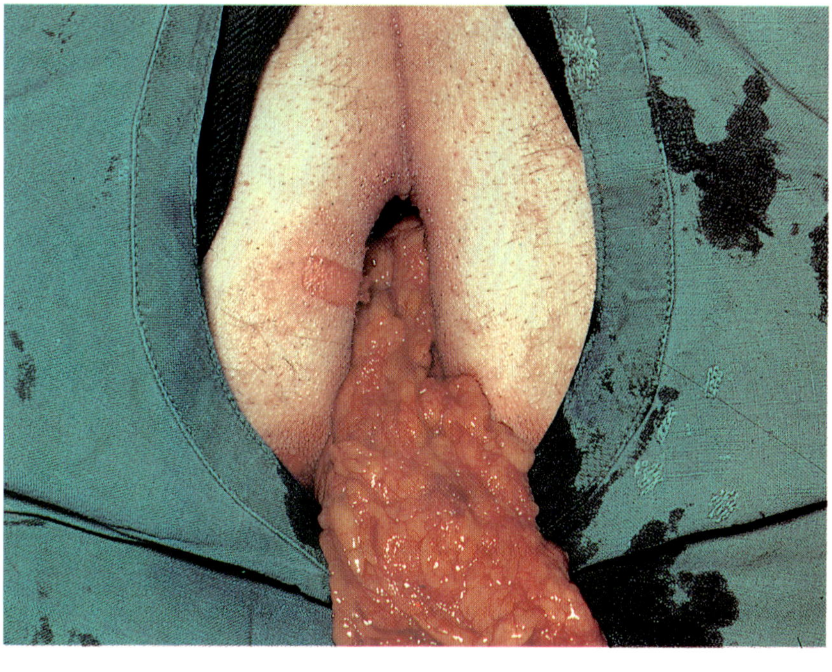

96 The same omentum brought down the left paracolic gutter and out through the perineal wound. Note how plentiful the omentum is, consequently being able to pack the pelvic cavity completely.

This male patient had fistulae necessitating wide skin excision around the anus. He had also lost a considerable amount of weight. Despite this a primary closure was achieved. In a patient with a colostomy the omentum will obliterate the lateral gap. In a procto-colectomy it will line the bared postero-lateral retroperitoneal wall.

97

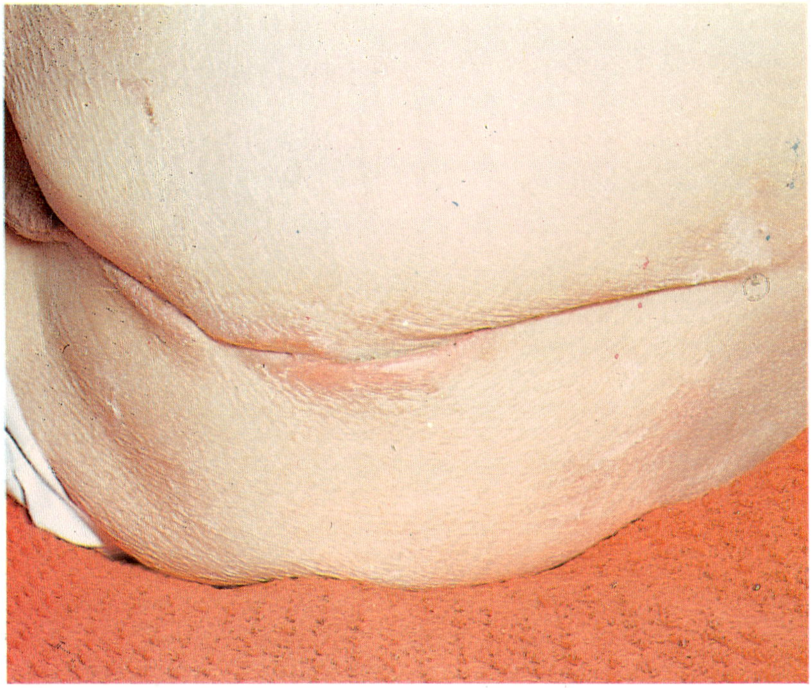

97 The same patient on the 16th post-operative day, just before discharge from hospital.

98

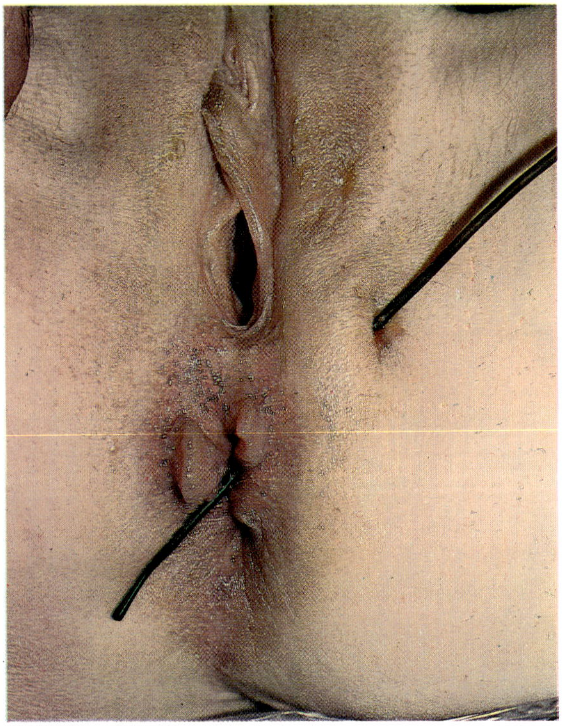

98 Widespread colonic Crohn's disease with anal involvement. If fistulae are neither deep nor extensive, and provided the main lesion is excised, curetting is adequate. In this patient, rectocolectomy was carried out with anal preservation, omental transplant and curettage of fistula. There was no involvement of the small bowel. A right iliac ileostomy was fashioned.

99

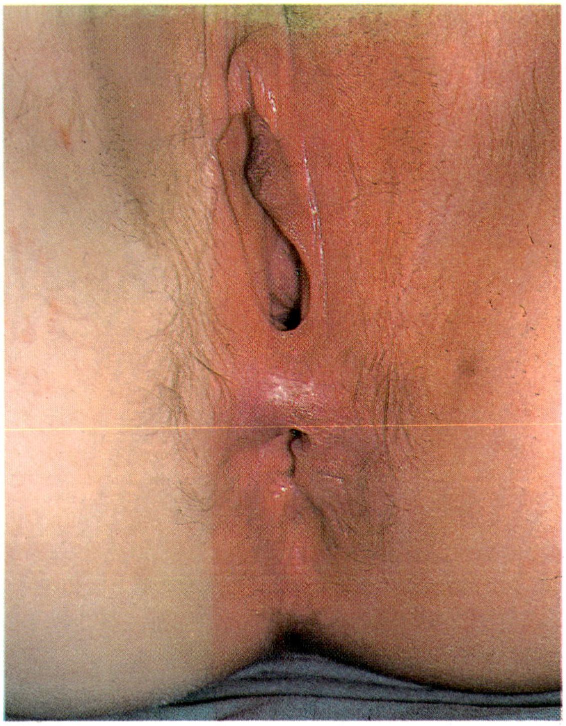

99 Same patient two months later. The anal closure healed by first intention. The swollen skin tags have disappeared and the curetted fistula has settled down completely.

The perineum has remained intact; and the patient admitted to no change in all aspects of sensory appreciation or motor contraction in that area.

X: THE ABDOMINAL INCISION

100

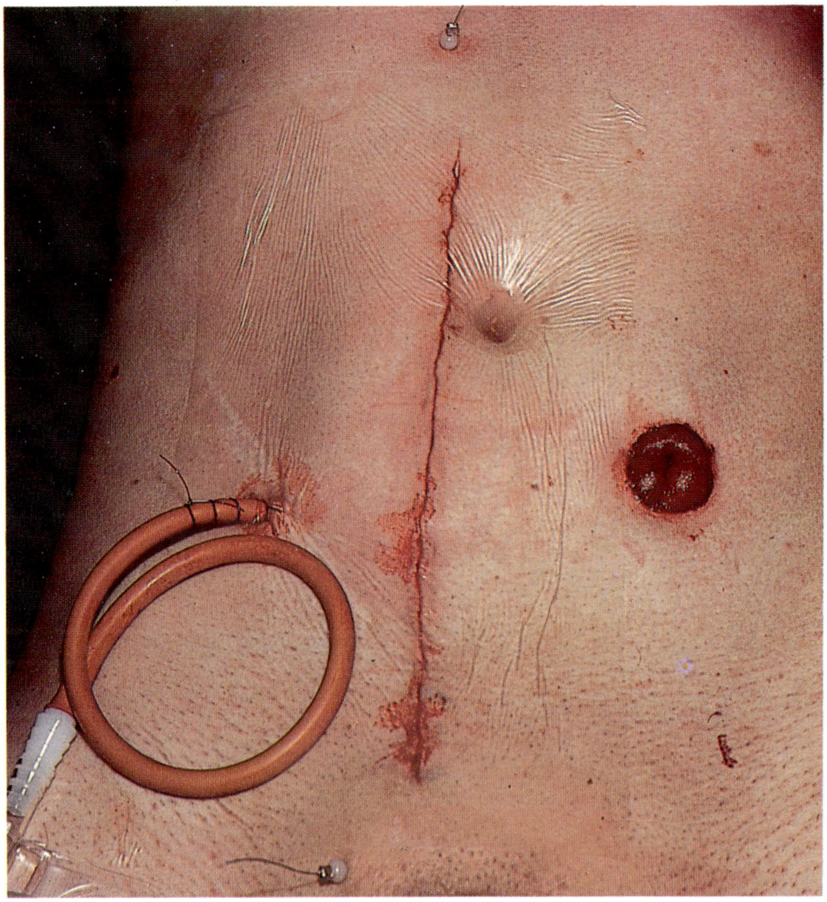

100 A right paramedian incision is preferable in a thin patient, though many surgeons use a midline incision, which leaves both iliac fossae free of scars. (Note the use of a subcuticular stitch held by beads (see Section III) to obtain a neat scar.)

101

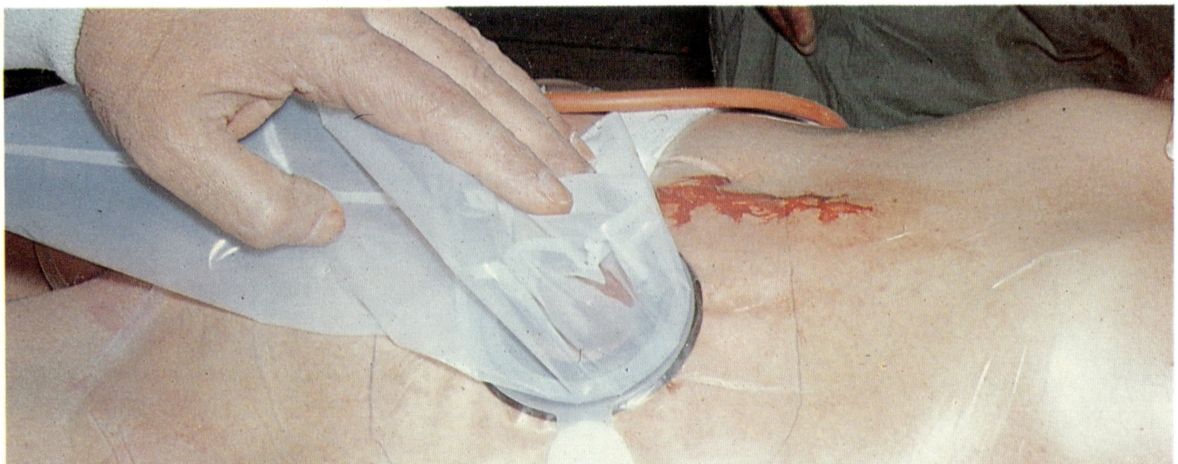

101 When correctly sited, the stoma lies midway between the waistline above and the hipline below. A light belt has been fitted to the appliance here to illustrate this point. The *wearing* of such a belt is not recommended.

102

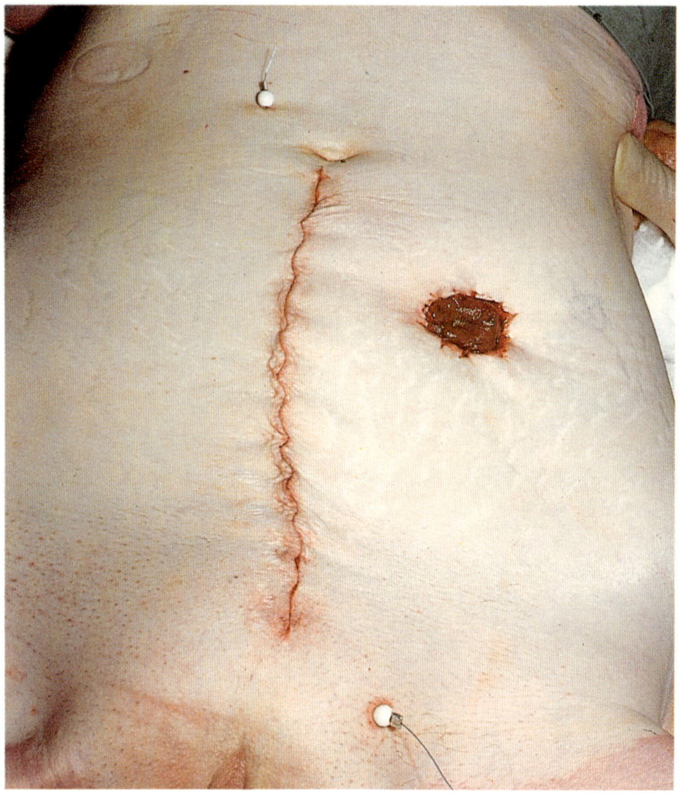

102 A midline incision in a thin patient. Such an incision works well in women as their wide pelvises leave ample room for the appliance.

103

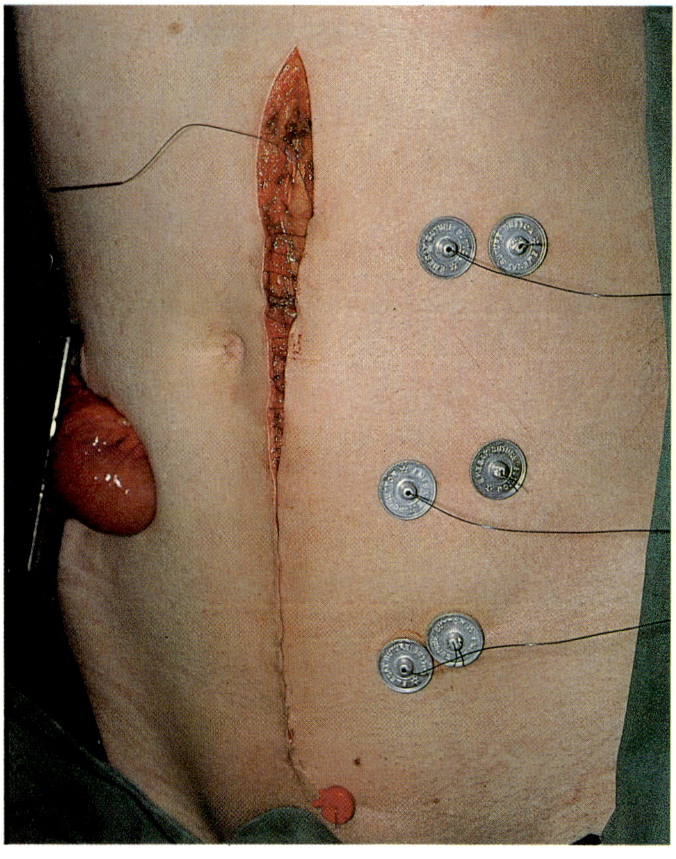

103 Total colectomy for ulcerative colitis in a poorly nourished patient. The incision is contralateral to the stoma. It must be sutured and sealed before the latter is fashioned. A subcuticular stitch (2/0 or 3/0 nylon) is the most elegant way of suturing the skin (shown here in its final stage of closure). It leaves a neater scar; reduces the incidence of suture abscesses; and its tension can be adjusted (see appendix) in the post-operative period thus reducing wound pain. If deep 'tension' sutures are used, they should be held on buttons *away* from the stoma so as not to interfere with the fitting of an appliance. Note that one end of each deep suture has not yet been crushed within the button, as the final correct tension is best gauged *after* the wound has been closed.

104

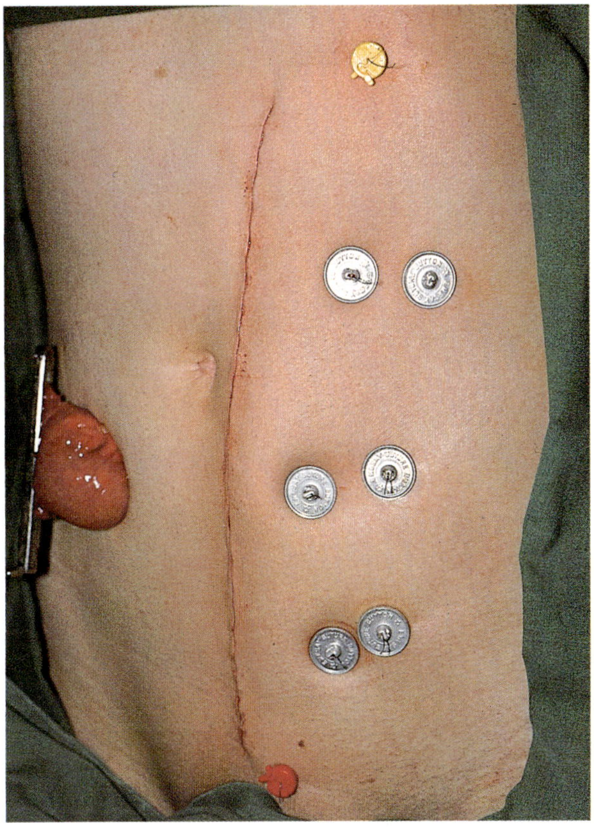

104 The completed wound closure. The subcuticular stitch is held on two plastic buttons (red and yellow) which can be opened to loosen or tighten the suture in the first post-operative days (see appendix).

If the 'tension' sutures have been correctly adjusted, their buttons should not indent the skin.

105

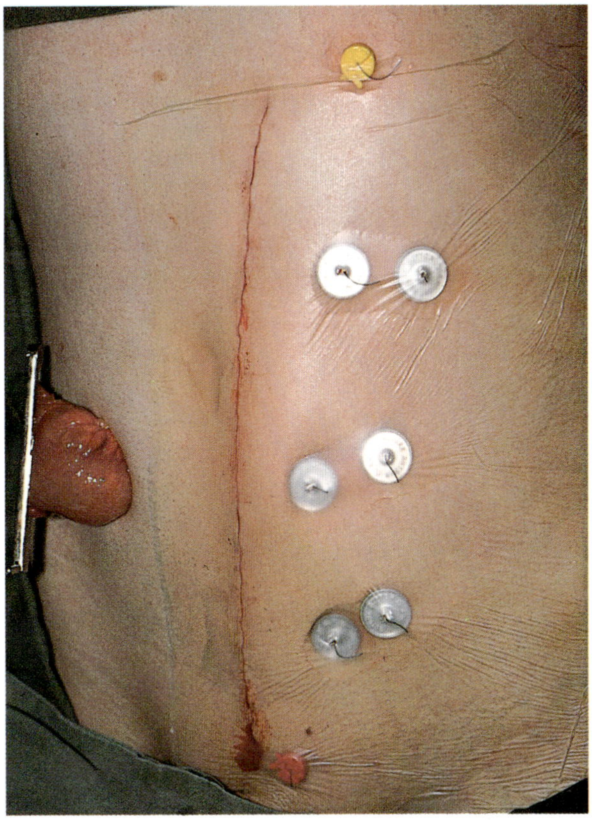

105 The wound and tension sutures are protected from any possible soiling from the stoma by sealing them over with a semi-permeable transparent drape that allows their frequent inspection without disturbance.

Note that the subcuticular stitch buttons lie at or beyond the edges of the drape. This allows the stitch to be removed about the tenth day without disturbing the drape or uncovering the wound. The stoma can now be unclamped in readiness for its muco-cutaneous suturing.

XI: SOME ABNORMAL STOMAS

106
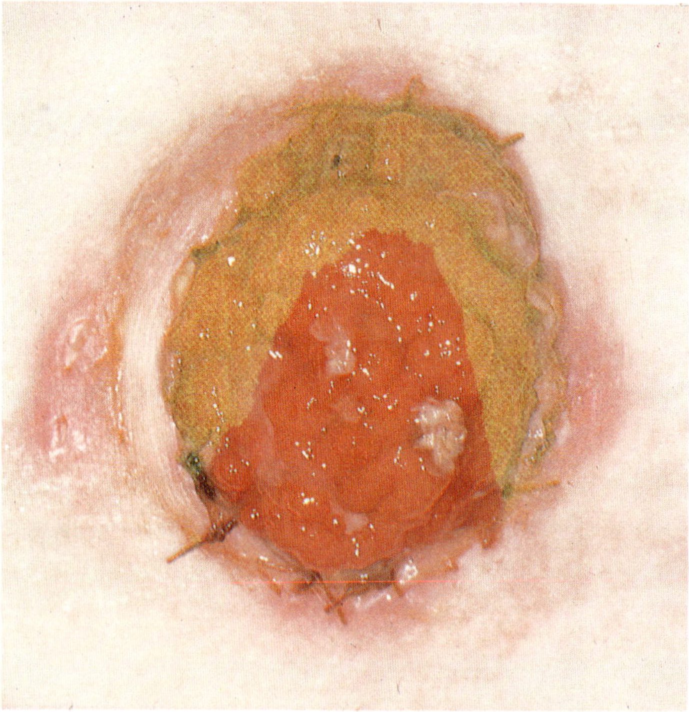

106 A colostomy performed in a patient presenting with obstruction from a carcinoma. It was not known before operation that he had polyposis coli!

107
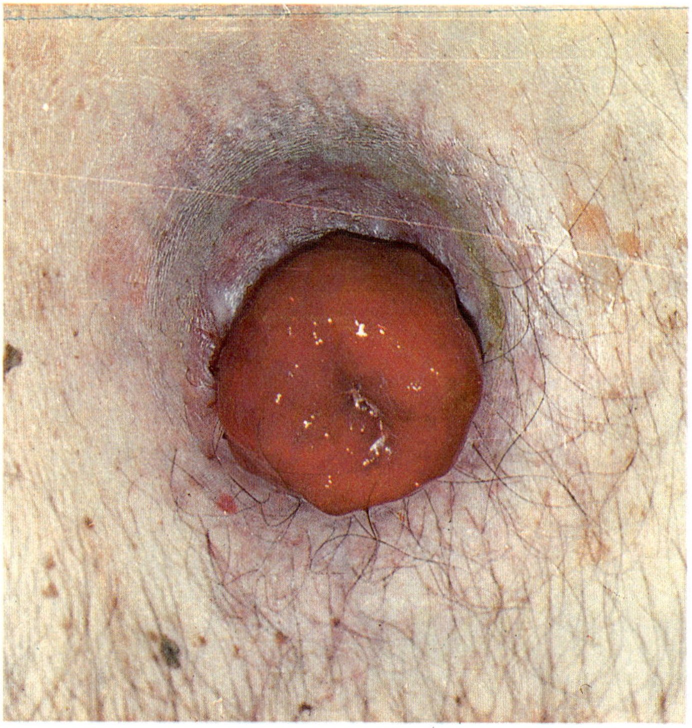

107 A colostomy in a patient with liver cirrhosis. Note the formation of a caput medusae. Bleeding from such varices can be troublesome and occasionally dangerous.

108

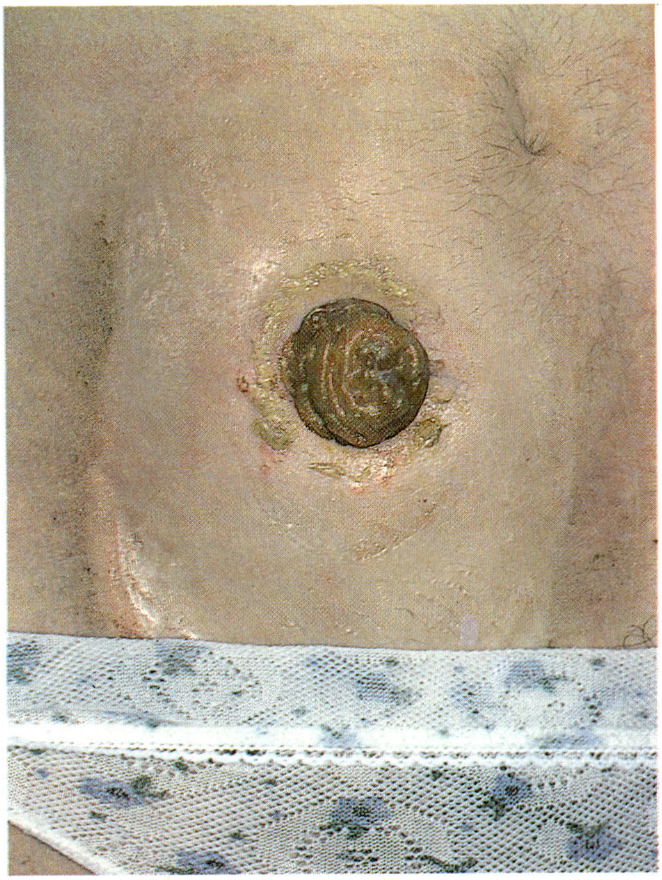

108 A young woman with a continent ileostomy of the Koch's type. The spout is on the proud side fostering mucus secretion and accumulation. It should preferably be a flush one.

109

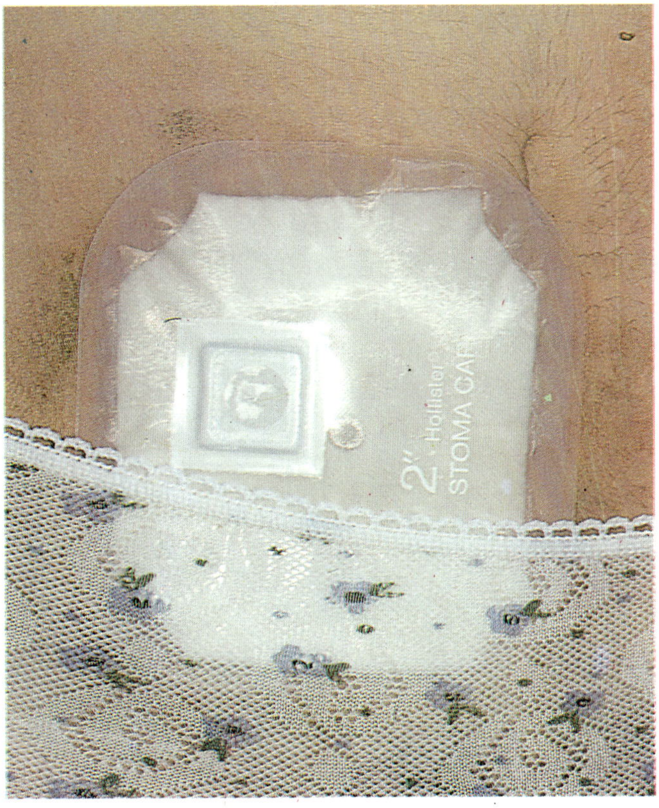

109 The same patient wearing a simple Hollister cap fitted with a filter. The latter is useful as gas can sometimes escape through a continent ileostomy.

110, 111, 112 A 'blow hole' fitted with a Biotrol magnetic appliance. One magnetic plate in the form of a washer adheres to the skin. The counter plate carries an obturator centrally pierced and fitted with a filter capped by a perforated plug.

110

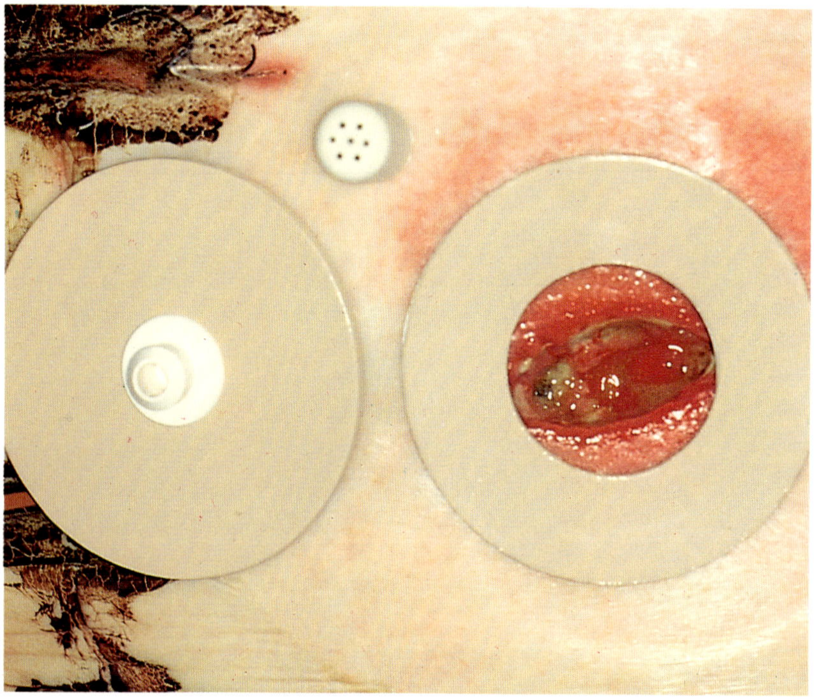

110 shows the three component parts of the appliance.

111

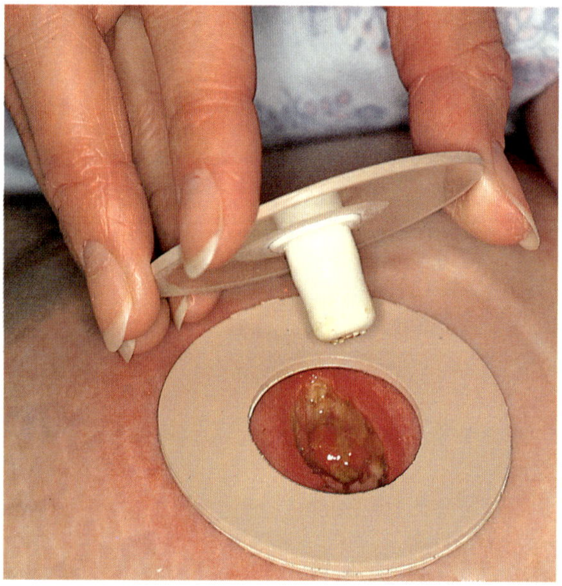

111 The perforated cap has been mounted on the obturator, and the two magnetic plates are being brought together.

112

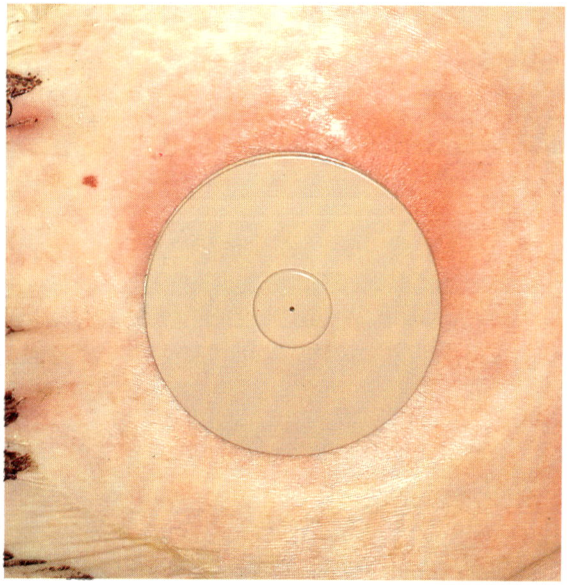

112 The appliance *in situ*.

113

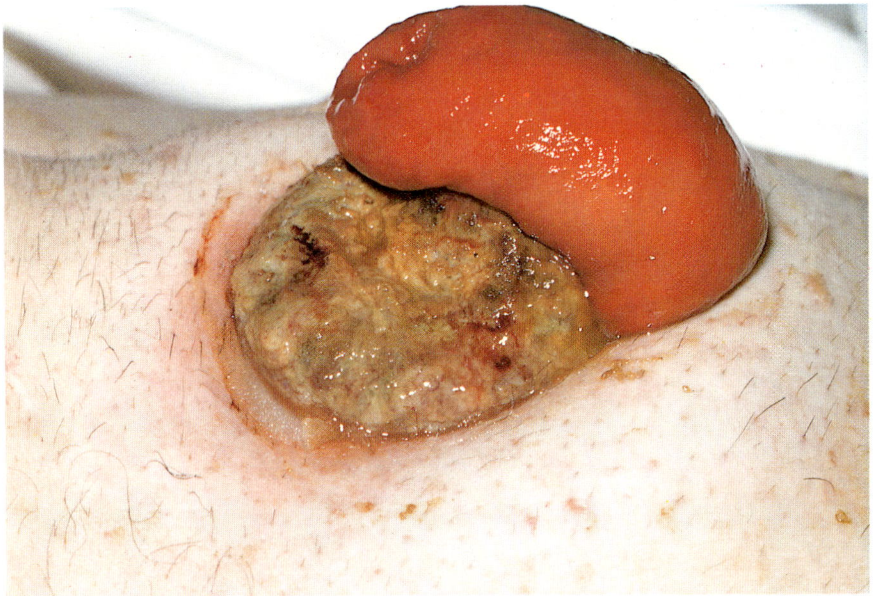

113 Ileostomy in a patient who underwent proctocolectomy for ulcerative colitis with a widespread carcinoma. The latter seeded in the ileostomy wound causing a fungating lesion interfering with the adhesive plate of the appliance.

114

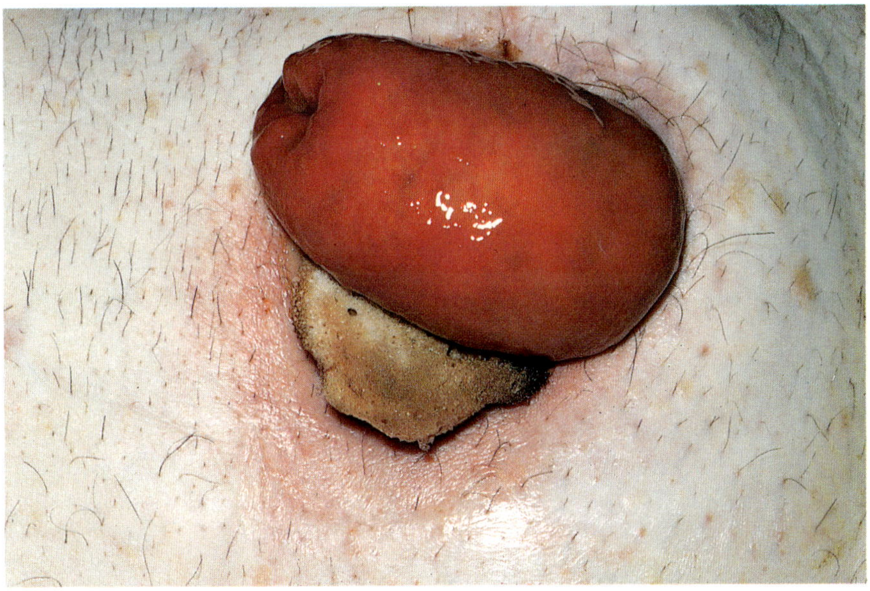

114 The lesion excised by a combination of diathermy and cryosurgery. The hole left by this procedure was filled with a silastic foam shaved back to the level of the skin so as not to interfere with the appliance.

115

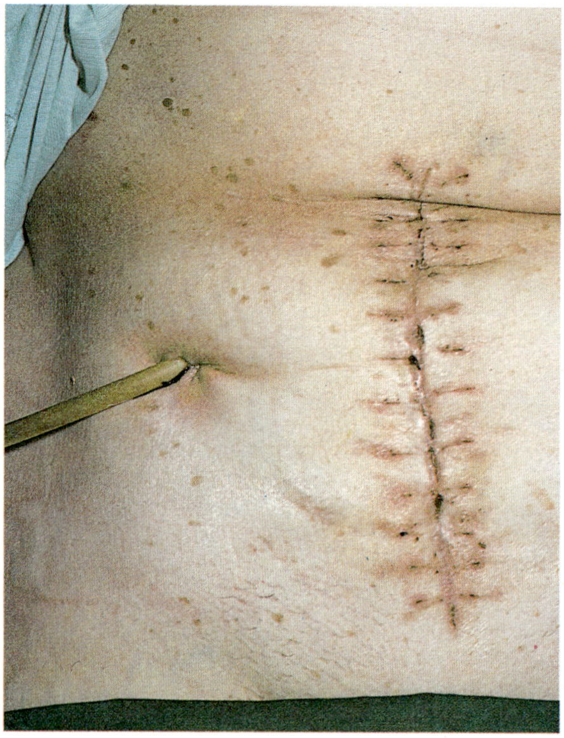

115 An 'insurance' tube caecostomy to protect an anastomosis. This procedure is unsatisfactory and is not recommended.

116

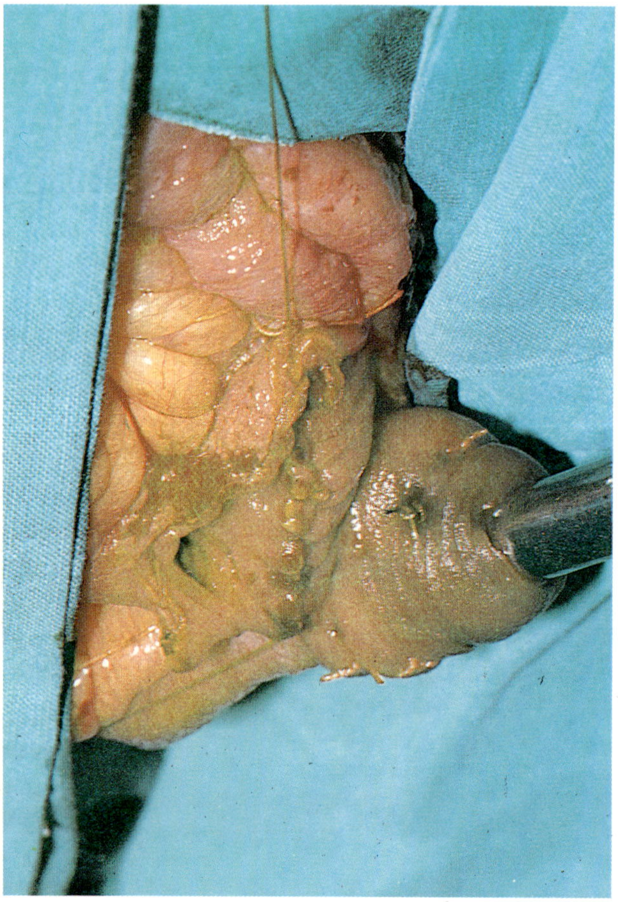

116 Construction of the 'valve' in a Koch's reservoir. The valve is the most important feature of the continent reservoir, and must be fashioned in a manner that will prevent it from unwrapping itself.

Here a Hegar dilator of suitable diameter is threaded through the valve and used as an anvil against which through-and-through non-absorbable sutures are inserted to hold together the intussuscepting loops of the valve. Note the incoming ileal loop to the right of the picture.

117

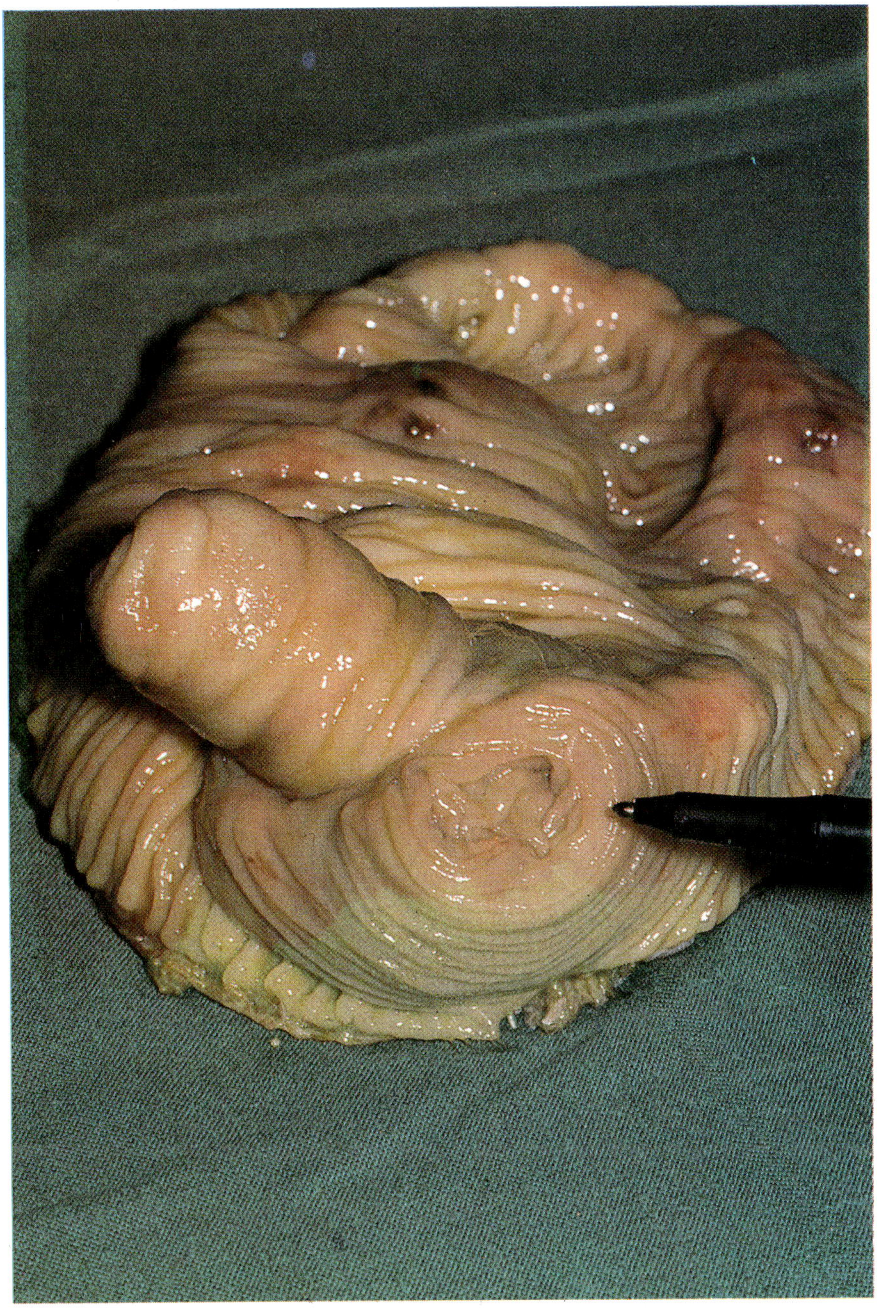

117 An excised specimen of a mature Koch's reservoir. The valve was still functioning and had remained straight. A pen points to the incoming ileal loop; the size of the reservoir can be appreciated.

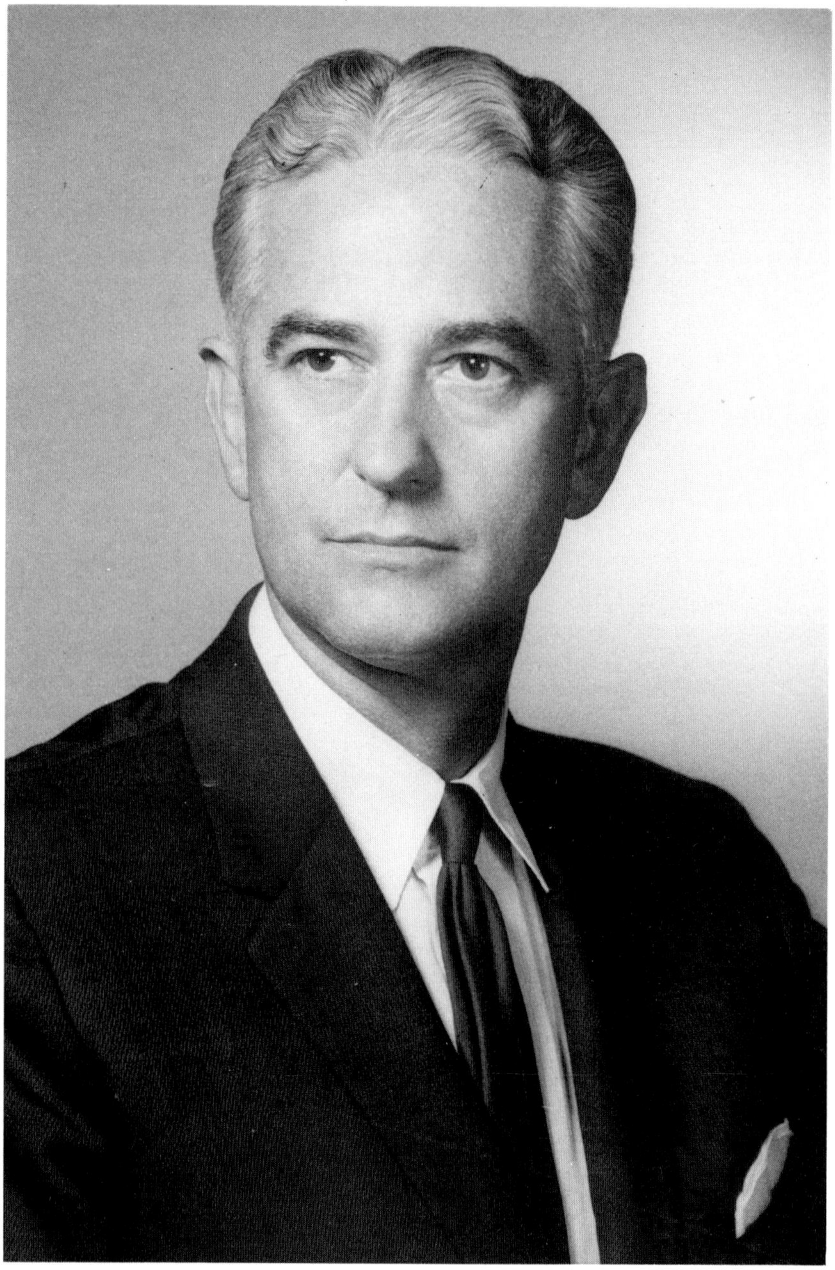

Rupert Beach Turnbull, Jr.
1913–1981
Father of stomatherapy

Section II Complications

XII: POOR SITING

118 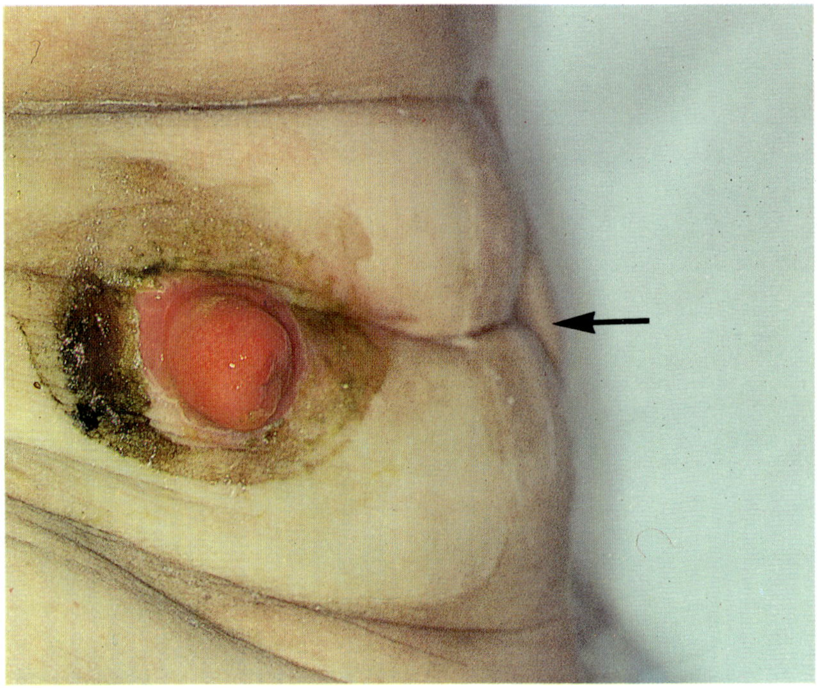

118 A badly sited ileostomy. Not only is it at the level of the umbilicus (arrowed), but it is crossed by a deep skin crease.

119 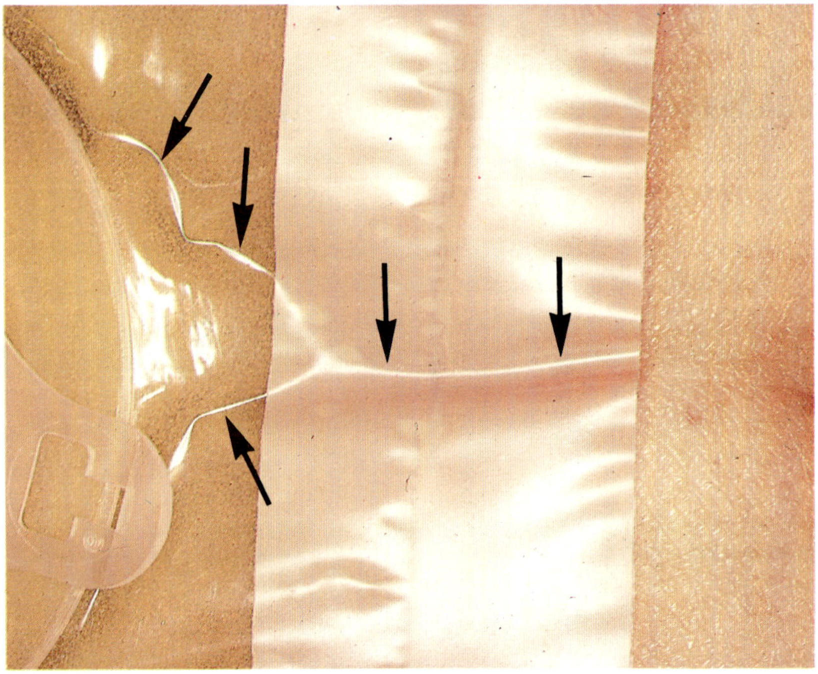

119 Shows how sitting, bending, etc., lifts off the adhesive plate from the skin even when held down further by an additional adhesive drape. The ileostomy effluents seeped under the raised areas (arrowed) and leaked at the level of the umbilicus.

Action required: Resite the ileostomy, or attempt a Z-plasty excising the fold. The latter was performed as it is the simpler method, and proved successful.

120

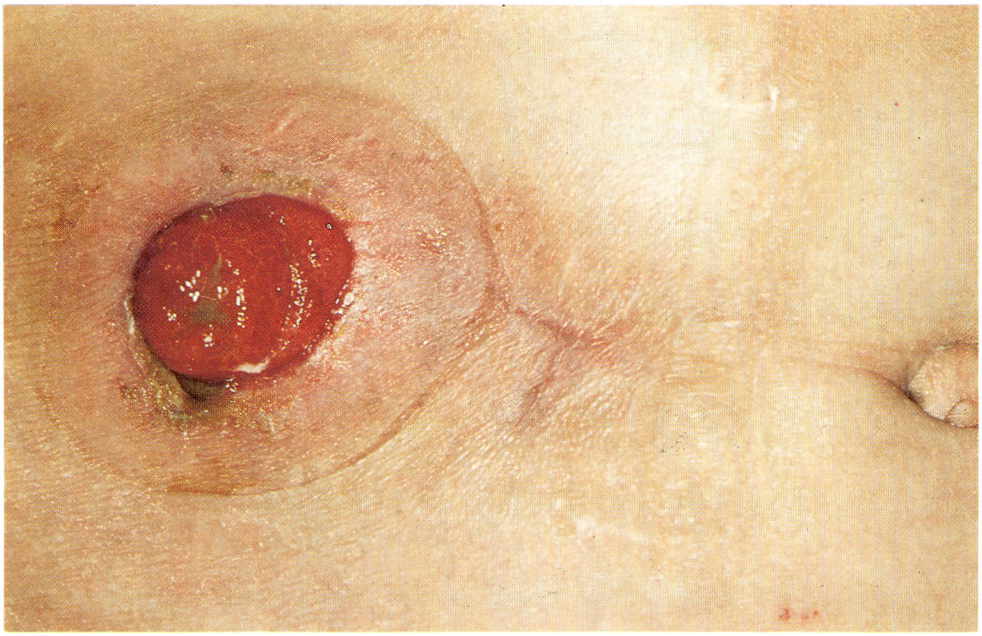

120 The post-operative situation. A close up view of the ileostomy area with the patient sitting. The previous skin crease has been ironed out, and the scar is well healed inspite of its close proximity to the stoma.

121

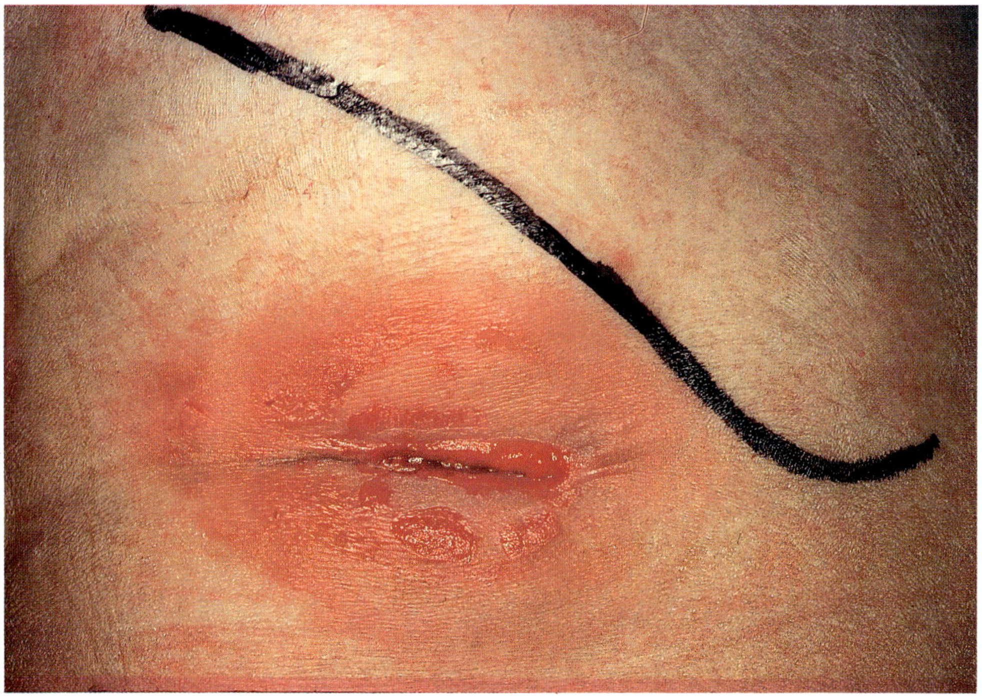

121 A disastrous site for a colostomy! The left transverse colon is not a suitable viscus for a colostomy. Its blood supply is suspect. It is not as mobile as the right transverse colon; and it lies at a deeper plane. The stoma is too close to the left subcostal margin, which interferes with the proper fitting of the appliance. The stoma has retracted and the peristomal skin has become ulcerated.

Action required: Protect skin immediately with karaya gum or Stomahesive (see appendix). Deal without delay with the lesions that necessitated the transverse colostomy, which should be closed. If this is not possible, refashion or resite it.

122
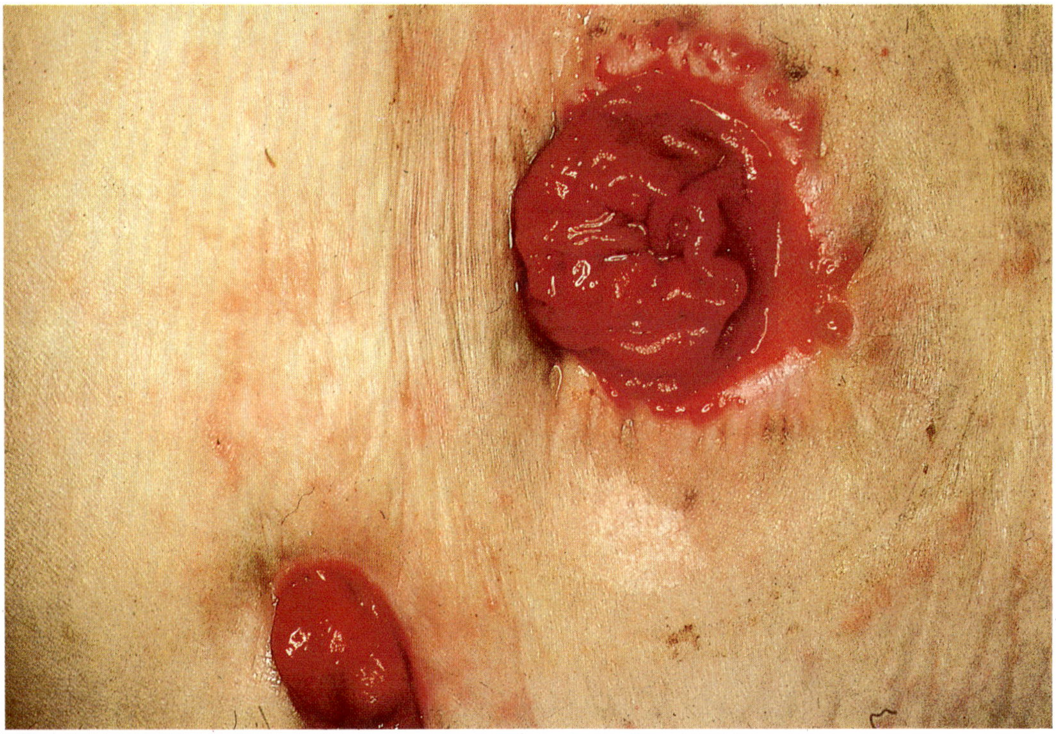

122 A badly sited mucus fistula. It is too close to the truly defunctioning left iliac colostomy and interferes with the adhesive plate of the appliance. It is best placed in the midline or to its right. Note the partial prolapse of the colostomy and the presence of muco-cutaneous granulomata.

123
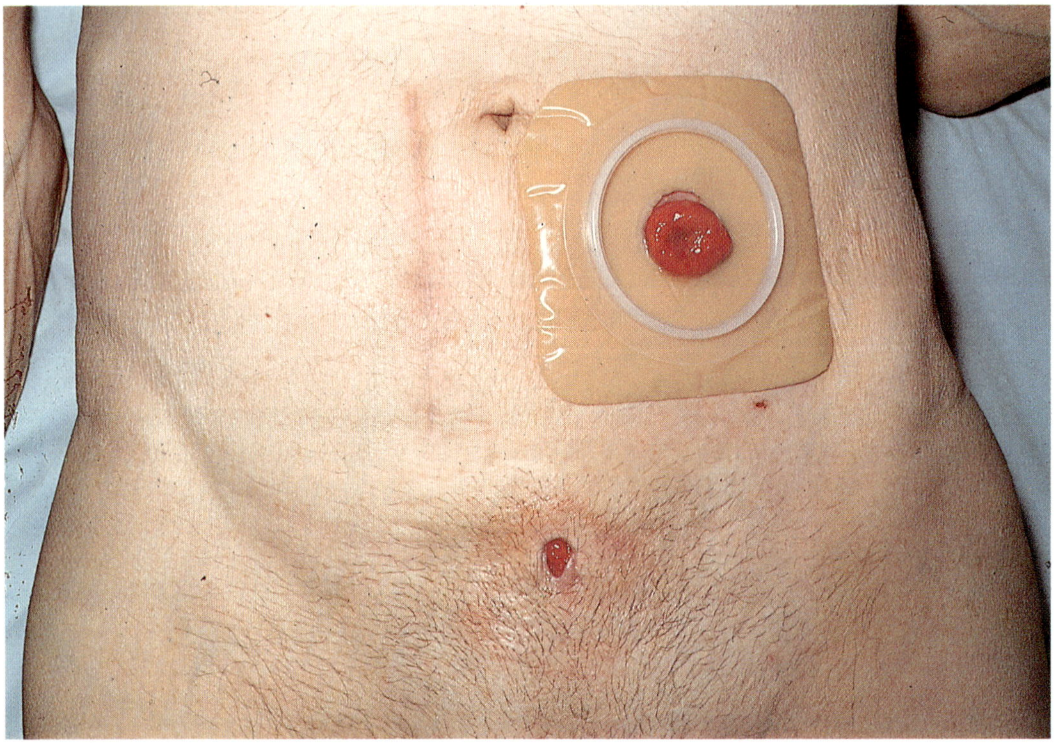

123 A good site for a mucus fistula. It is well away from the appliance and the incision (note advantage of latter on the contralateral side), and in the midline. It would be even better if it were higher up, above the pubic hairline.

124

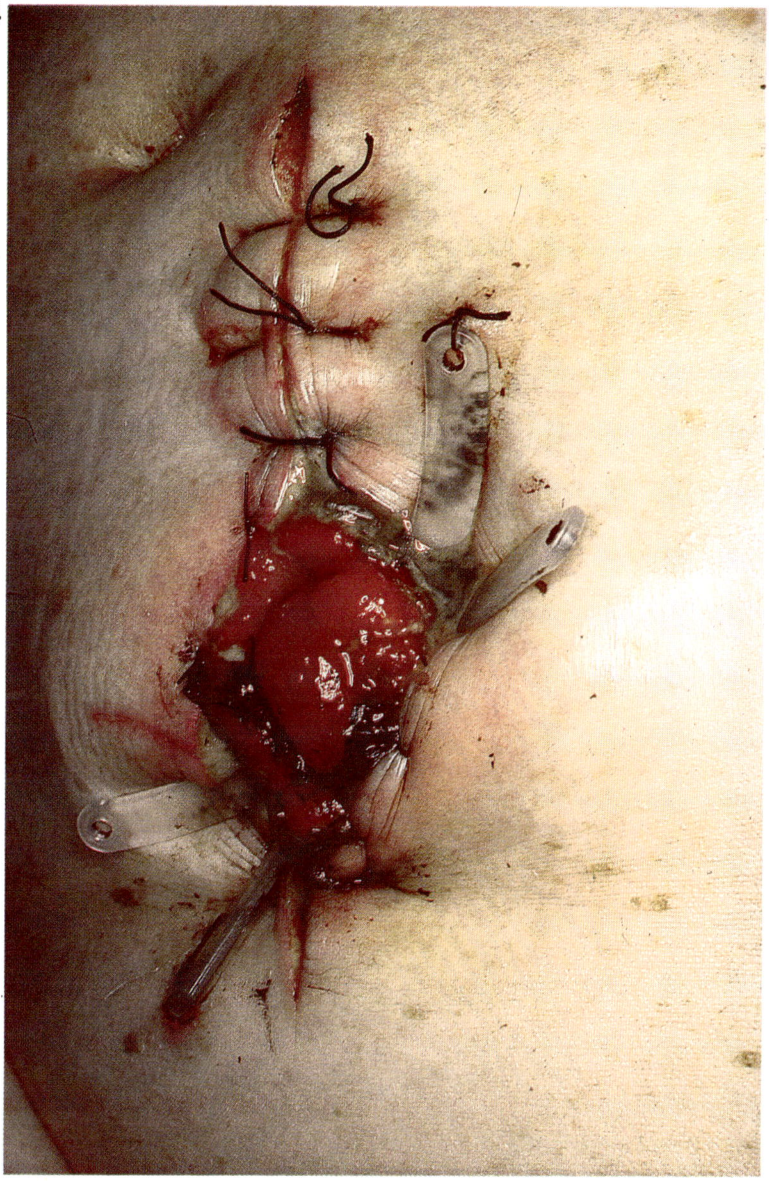

124 A catastrophic site. The lower sigmoid colon is not a suitable site for a colostomy.

A defunctioning loop colostomy fashioned in the lower sigmoid colon has been sited at the inferior end of a poorly sutured left lower paramedian incision, and held in position by means of a plastic cross. No appliance could be fitted to this colostomy, as the plastic cross, the poorly sutured incision, and above all the symphysis pubis interfered with its adhesive plate.

When the plastic cross was removed, tension on the colon caused the colostomy to retract and disappear.

XIII: STOMA PROPER

The stoma proper

Necrosis — limited / extensive

Retraction — early / late — partial / total

Prolapse — partial / total

Bleeding see Chapter XIV

Necrosis

The normal stoma in the immediate post-operative days is plum coloured and shiny. When necrosis or gangrene occurs, the mucosa becomes black and loses its shine. In a colostomy this is caused by an impaired vascular supply from the marginal artery of the middle colic. In an ileostomy – usually in obese people – it follows damage to the post-arcade terminal arteries.

Limited necrosis. This affects only a quadrant of the stoma, often anti-mesenteric; or the distal centimetre or so of the stoma.

Management. Leave alone and watch. The mucosa will slough; granulation tissue will form, and may epithialise to produce an acceptable stoma.

If epithialisation does not take place, the stoma should be excised early and refashioned.

If fibrosis results, it may be partial, affecting only the quadrant involved, with distortion of the stoma. If this interferes with the appliance, refashion it. If fibrosis is total and forms a fibrous stenotic ring, excise and refashion the stoma.

Extensive necrosis. This can only be determined by endoscopy with a thin sigmoidoscope or proctoscope. Several centimetres are affected with intraperitoneal bowel death. It is due to damage to a main artery and is uncommon.

Management. Immediate laparotomy; further bowel mobilisation, and establishment of a new and fully viable stoma.

Either type can be a complication of a neglected acute prolapse necessitating the excision of the necrotic exteriorised gut.

125

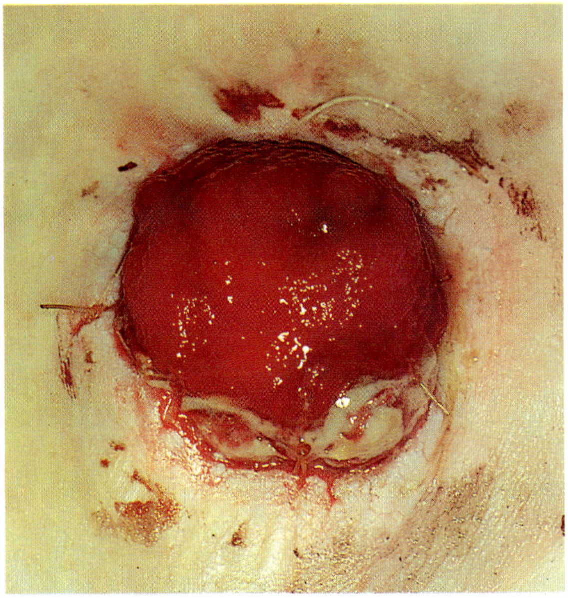

126

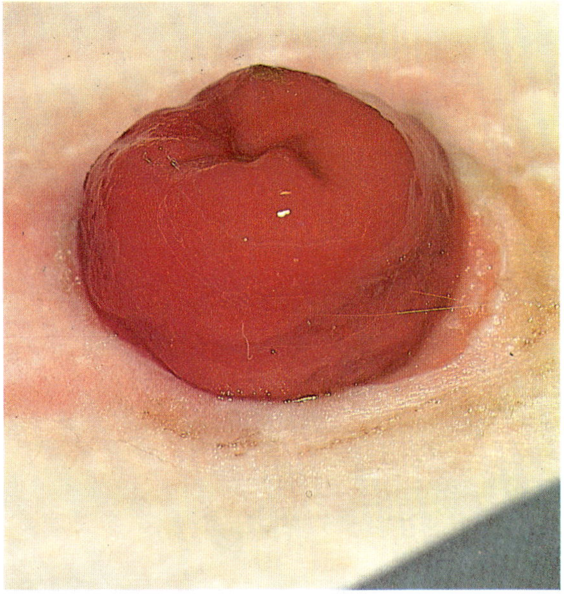

125 Partial necrosis at the anti-mesenteric border, during the first post-operative week, in an ill-nourished patient with Crohn's disease.

The lesion was treated conservatively and watched. Sloughing took place with formation of granulation tissue and epithialisation.

126 Three months later, after careful stoma care, constant guidance, adequate protein intake and repeated reassurance, a very good result was obtained.

127

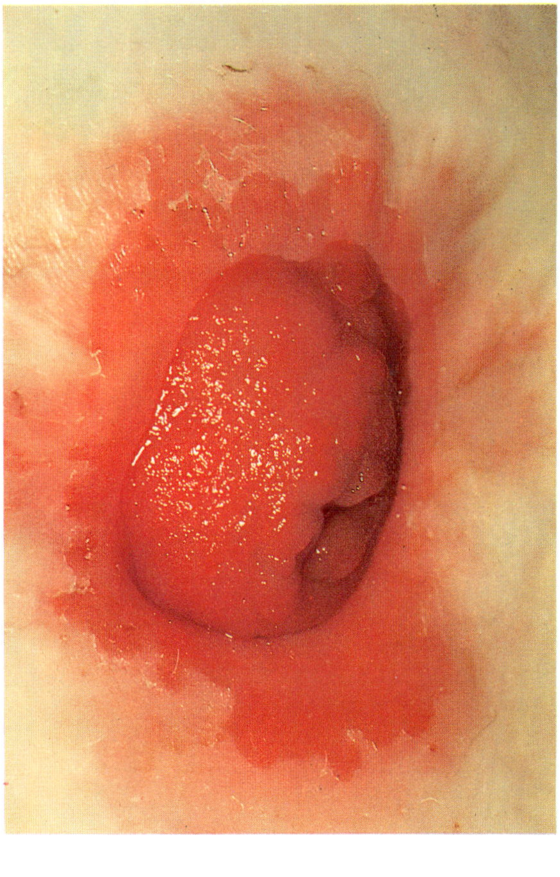

127 A similar case of necrosis; but here, despite active stoma care, scarring took place and led to the distortion of the stoma with poor fitting of the appliance and peri-stomal excoriation. The submucosa and part of the muscle coat had probably not survived.

The stoma was reconstructed.

128

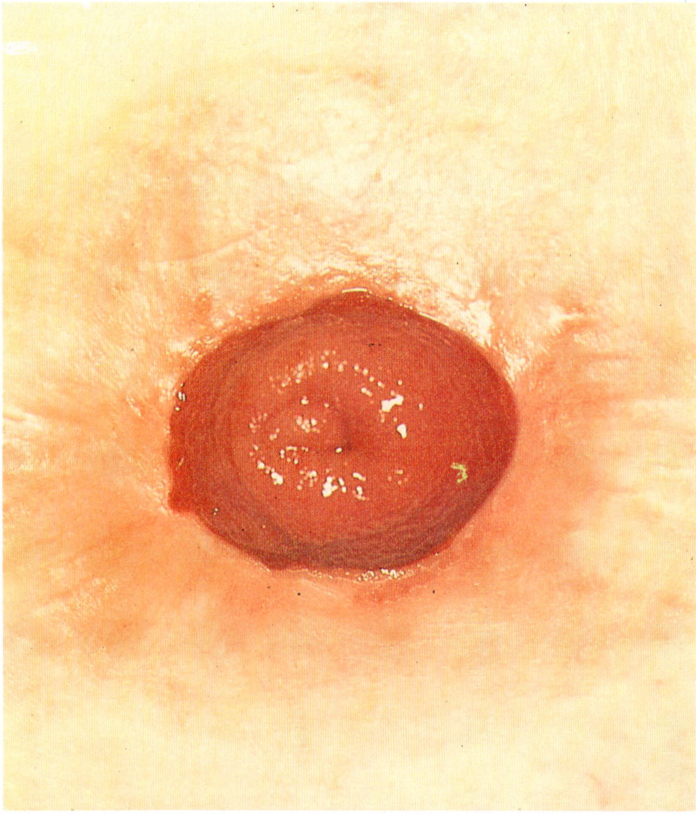

128 The stoma three months after refashioning.

129

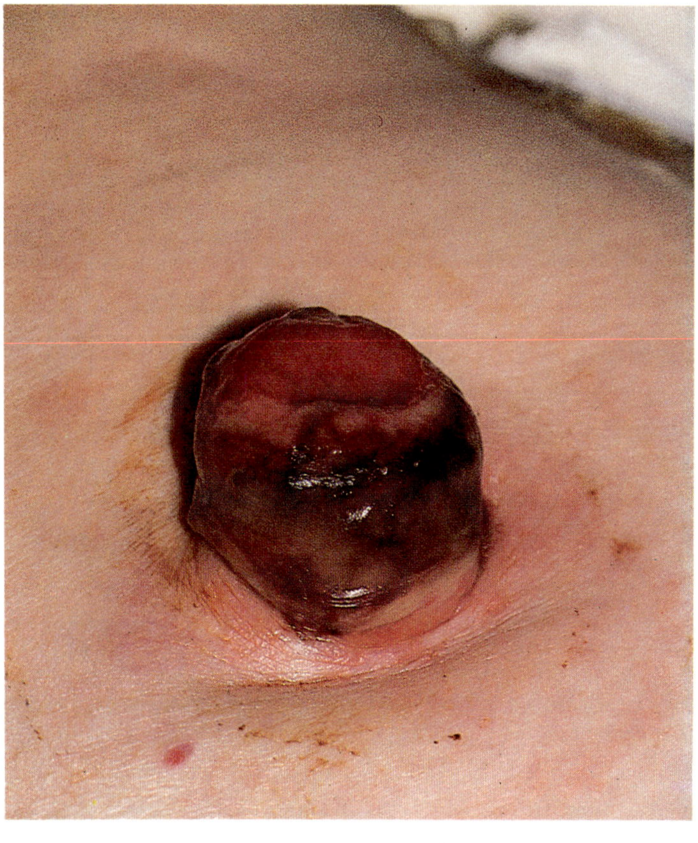

129 Necrosis of most of the mucosa of the returning coat of a colostomy. Although extensive, it was treated conservatively and carefully watched. The mucosa separated, but the submucosa and underlying muscle layers survived. Complete re-epithialisation followed.

130

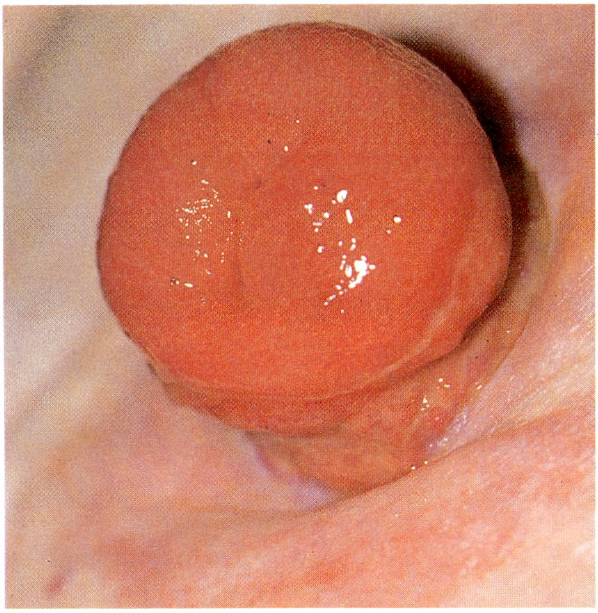

130 The same colostomy five weeks later. A clear mucosal border can be seen advancing over a healthy and well vascularised submucosa.

131

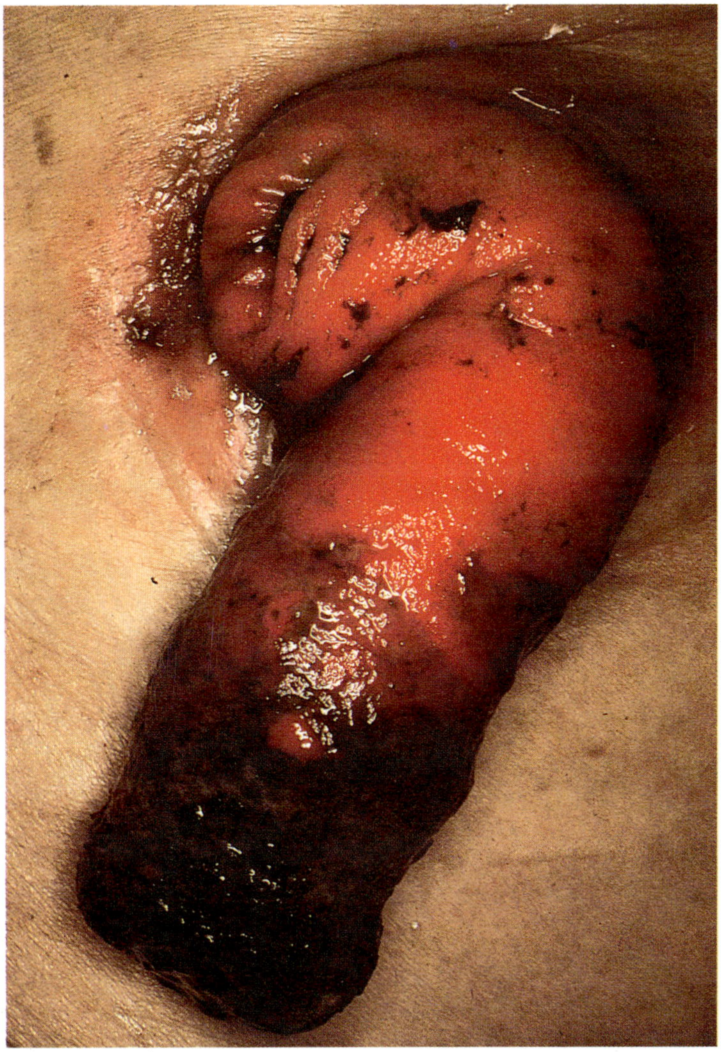

131 A neglected acute prolapse of the distal limb of a transverse colostomy. The resulting retrograde intussusception led to interference with the blood supply and caused gangrene of the leading end.

Action required: The underlying disease should be dealt with and the colostomy closed. If this is impracticable, it should be converted to separate barrels.

Retraction

Retraction can be:

(a) Early – while the patient is still in hospital.

(b) Late – months to years later.

It can be partial or total; fixed or intermittent.

Early retraction

- occurs in the post-operative period, more frequently in the obese.
- it is due to tension on the colostomy.
- it can be anticipated or prevented by supporting the mesentery over a thin glass rod.
- will be followed by a ring of granulation tissue, and does not need urgent interference.
- can be watched, as many will give a satisfactory stoma.
- may be a nuisance, specially in ileostomy, inducing leakage and skin excoriation.
- if skin problems arise, or stenosis ensues, refashion.

Late retraction

- can result from gross increase in body weight post-operatively, due to increasing thickness of subcutaneous fat. Invite patient to diet.
- may result from herniation if the trephine hole was too large.
- may occur in transverse colostomy if rod has been removed too early and the loop undergoes recession.

Fixed retraction will result from most of the above, and if it cannot be managed successfully by careful stoma care, reconstruction – usually local – is required.

Intermittent retraction is more common in ileostomies than colostomies. It is a failure of fixation of the everted bowel; the stoma retracts when the patient is recumbent, and reappears when he stands up. It can lead to leakage and skin soreness. The fault is inadequate fixation of the gut to the anterior abdominal wall or rectus sheath during stoma construction, and the use of absorbable suture for this purpose.

132

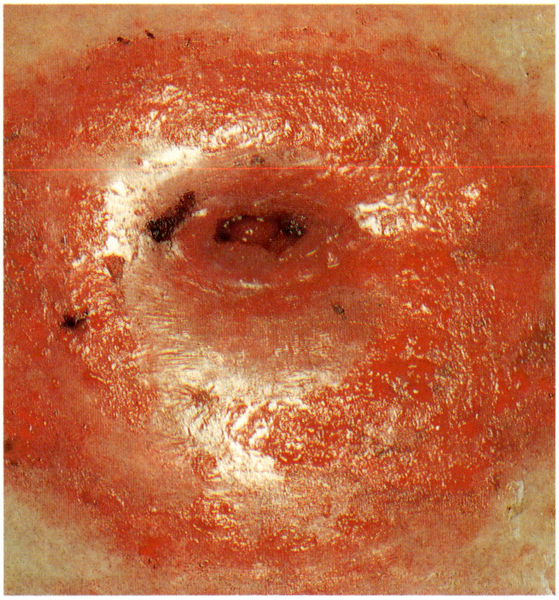

132 Early retraction in a transverse colostomy, with severe skin excoriation due to the high enzyme content of faeces.

Action required: Deal with main lesion and close colostomy. If not possible, refashion immediately.

133

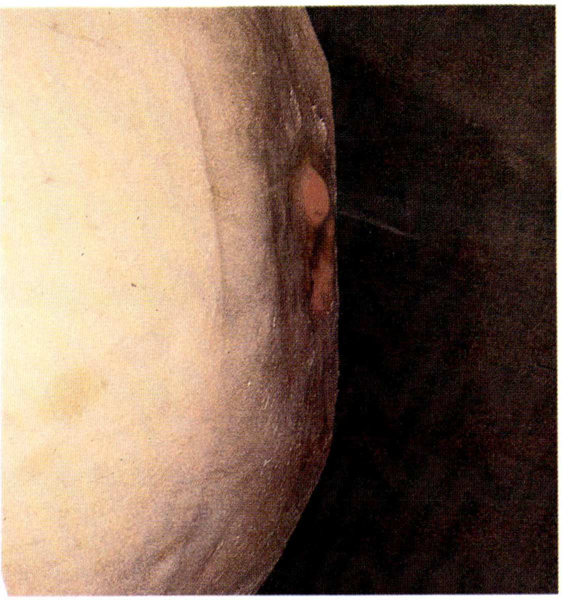

134

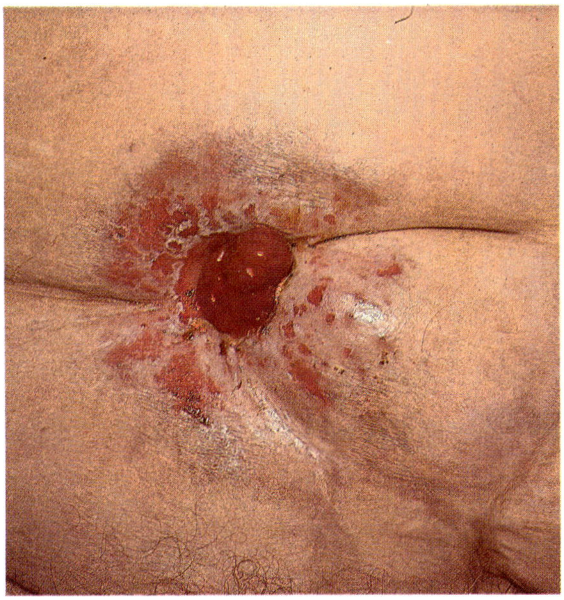

133 Late retraction of an ileostomy due to herniation.

Action required: Repair hernia; if not likely to be successful, transplant ileostomy to another site.

134 Late retraction in a patient who put on weight and developed thick skin folds, 15 years after the ileostomy. The patient could no longer wear an appliance and became a recluse. Note that the ileostomy was too close to umbilicus.

The ileostomy was transplanted to a more suitable site that was more accessible to the patient.

135

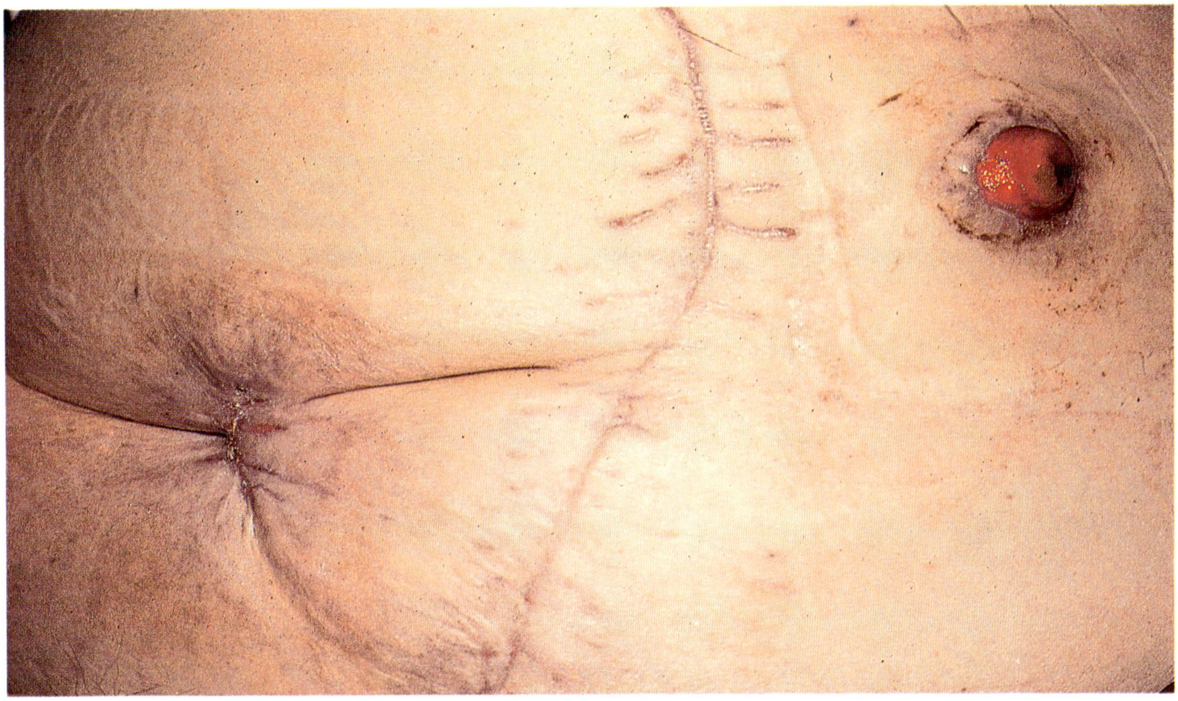

135 Two weeks after transplantation to the left upper abdominal quadrant.

136 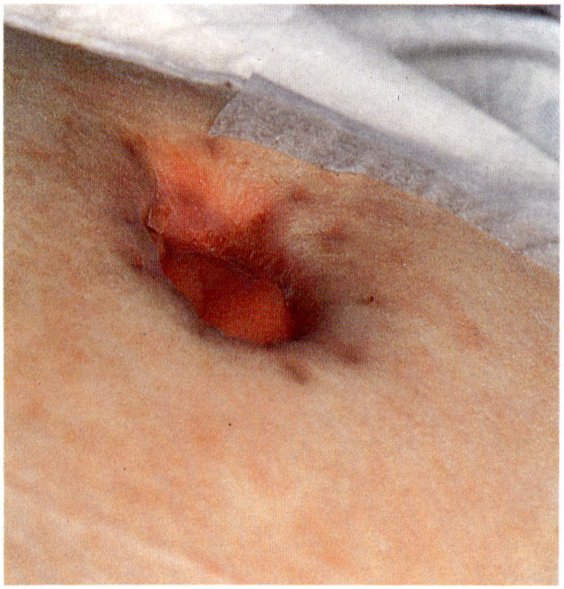

136 Not all retractions are troublesome. This one occurred in an elderly patient early after surgery; but the patient's stools were well formed, and were evacuated twice a day causing him no problems.

Action required: Leave well alone!

Prolapse

Prolapse can be partial or total. It is generally fixed (or chronic) but can be intermittent.

Occasionally an unusual rise in intra-abdominal pressure can cause an acute prolapse which should be reduced immediately to avoid circulatory difficulties. This manoeuvre can be undertaken under intravenous diazepam sedation. If unsuccessful, surgical reduction should be carried out.

Prolapse is common in transverse colostomy, and involves either the distal loop by reverse intussusception, or both loops. It is not uncommon in ileostomy, but is comparatively rare in end colostomy.

Prevention techniques:

- good closure of the lateral space using unabsorbable suture, attaching the cut posterior and lateral peritoneal edges to the mesentery of the colon or ileum, right up to the trephine hole.
- building spouts of the correct lengths; too long a spout inviting prolapse.
- using a trephine hole of the correct size: too large an aperture engenders prolapse.

Management strategies:

- Small or partial ones or those complicating a temporary stoma do not usually need interference.
- When pronounced or total, refashion if it interferes with appliance management. Recurrence is not uncommon and may need repeated refashioning.
- If fault is due to too large an aperture, reducing it by suturing may prove unsuccessful. Resiting is then required.

Note: Colostomies, and more specially ileostomies, may vary in length over the course of the day according to the peristaltic activity of the gut. This is the normal state and should not be mistaken for an intermittent prolapse.

137

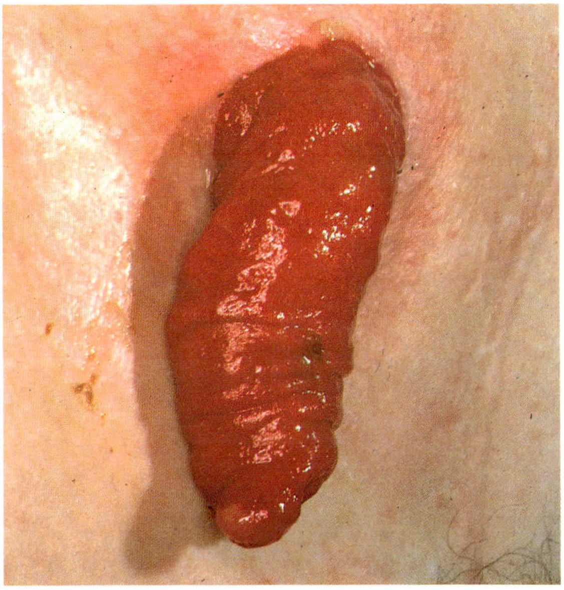

137 A total ileostomy prolapse of static length. It did not worry the patient, and did not interfere with the appliance, which was specially chosen to prevent trauma of inferior muco-cutaneous edge of stoma. No reconstruction was needed.

138

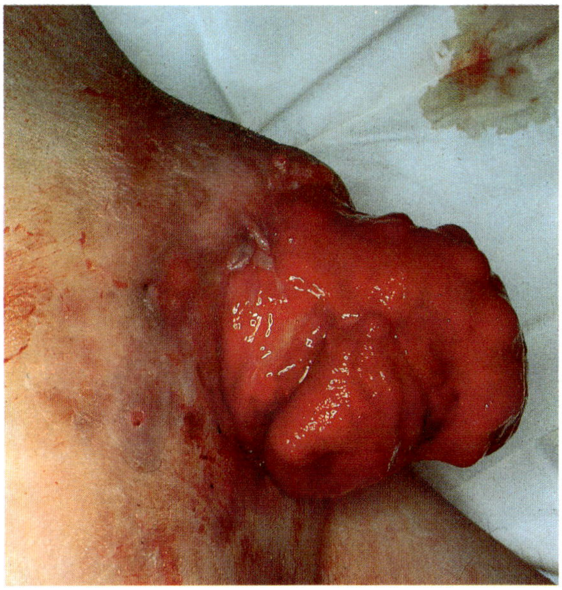

138 Prolapse of both loops of a transverse colostomy, complicated by herniation. The appliance fitted poorly, resulting in small skin ulcers and granulomata. The prolapse was caused by too big an opening in the abdominal wall and inadequate right lateral fixation of the short transverse colonic loop.

Action required: Apply a protective wafer to the skin while preparing the patient for definitive surgery to the causative disease; close the colostomy at the same time. If definitive surgery is contra-indicated, refashion or resite the colostomy.

139

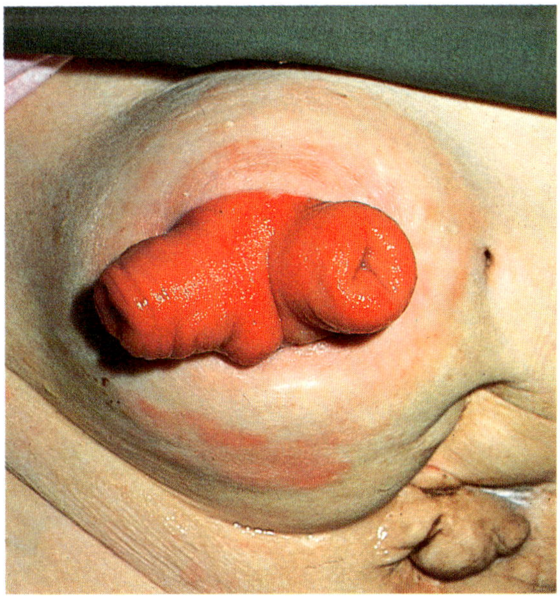

139 A similar problem to that in **138**. Resection was contra-indicated. Conversion to split barrels was therefore chosen. Careful stoma care produced healthy peri-stomal skin that enhanced the successful outcome of conversion.

140

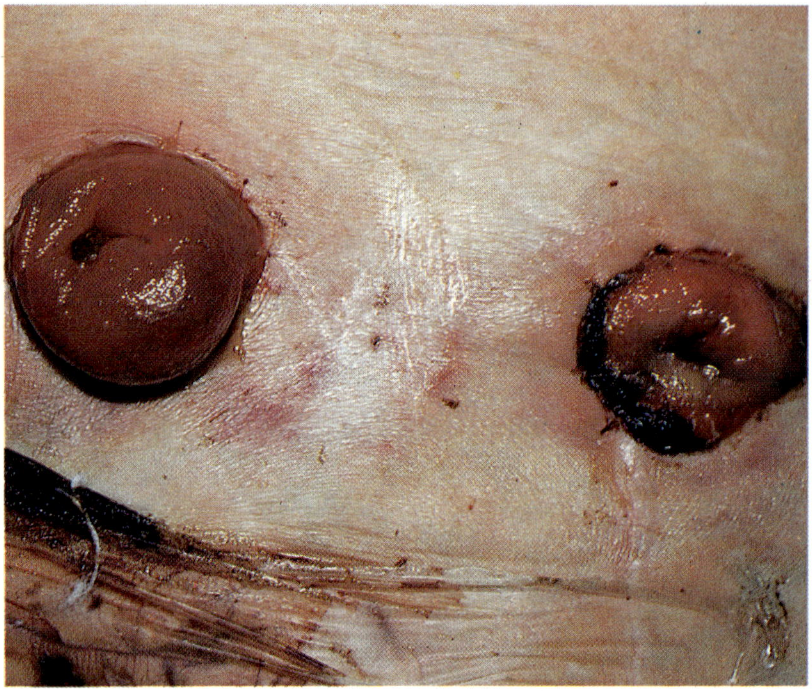

140 The same patient, a week after conversion to split barrels.

141

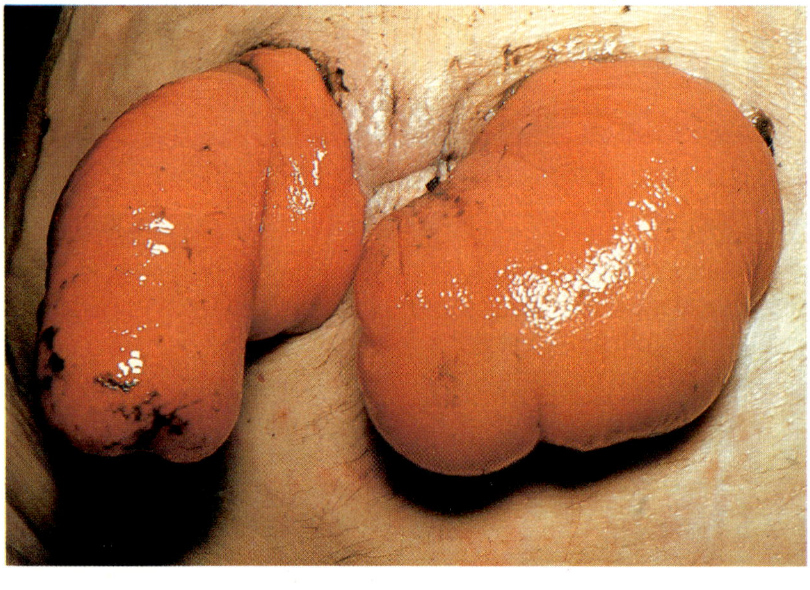

141 Prolapse in both limbs of a split barrel colostomy. The latter is a truly defunctioning colostomy and was used here to rest the colon in a case of severe diverticulitis. The prolapses caused little inconvenience and, after sigmoidectomy, normal transverse colonic continuity was restored.

142

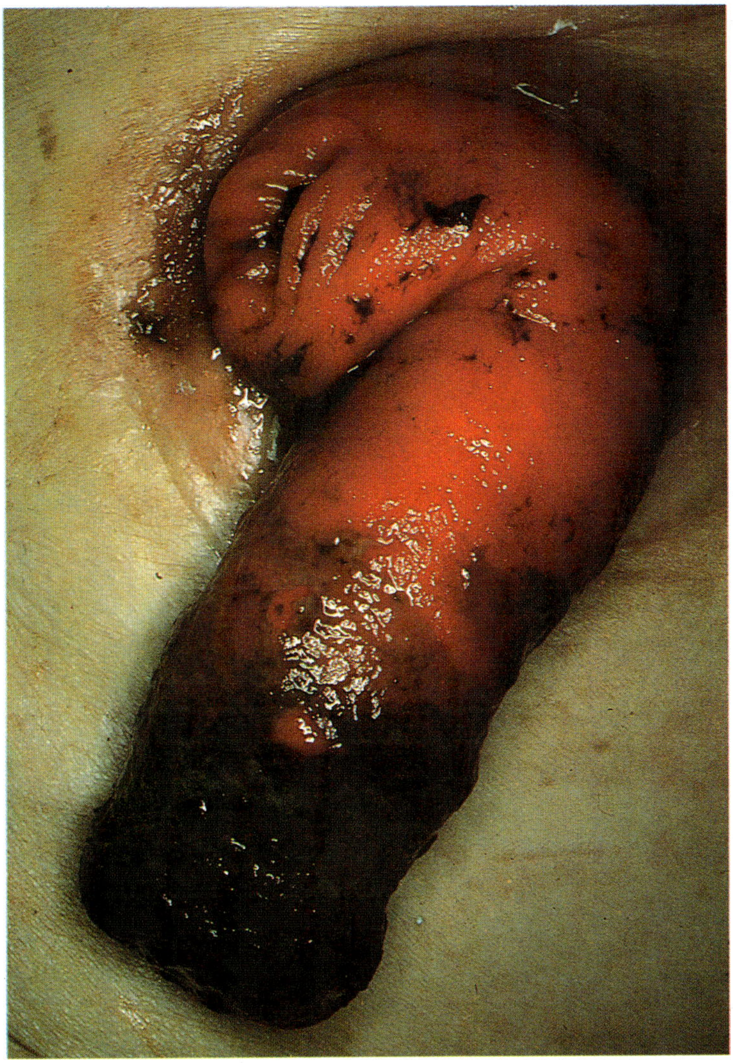

142 Acute prolapse in a transverse colostomy. The delay in reduction led to gangrene in its leading end. (Same case as **131**.)

Action required: Deal with the causative disease urgently and close the colostomy at the same time. If this is not possible, convert it to separate barrels after total excision of the prolapse.

143

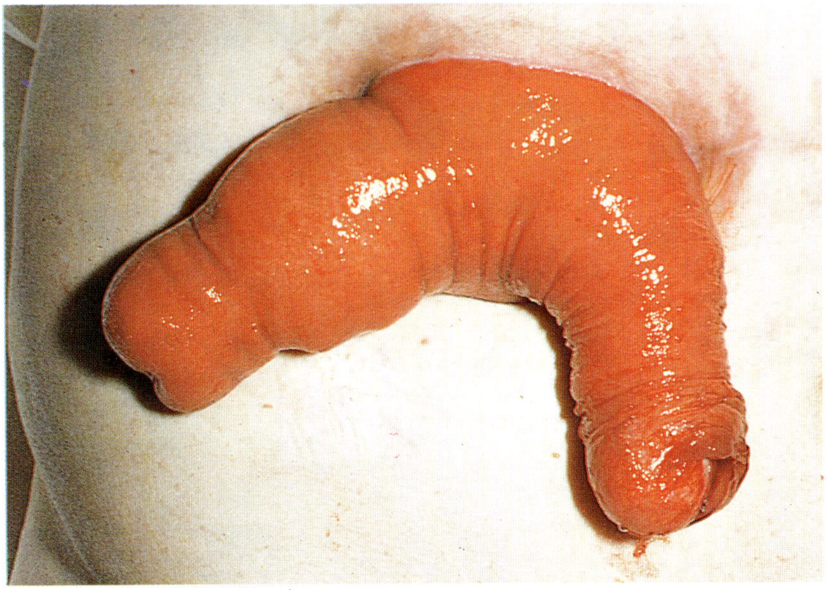

143. A transverse colostomy in a transverse exploratory incision. Too wide an opening was left at one side of the wound. Within two weeks of surgery a double prolapse had occurred. The problem was further complicated by ascites.

Massive liver secondaries were present and the patient died shortly afterwards.

XIV: MUCO-CUTANEOUS JUNCTION

The muco-cutaneous junction

- Bleeding
- Detachment
  - partial
  - total
- Fistula
  - superficial
  - deep
- Pyogenic granulomata
- Stenosis

Bleeding

If post-operative haemorrhage occurs it is usually during the first 48 hours following surgery and is rarely severe. It differs from the expected thin bloodstained serous fluid in the bag – clots appearing at the muco-cutaneous junction, or alongside the appliance ring.

Oozing. This is usually venous or capillary in origin. On removing the appliance it appears as a slowly-forming pool in one of the quadrants of the stoma. It usually comes from the edge of the gut.

It should be treated conservatively by wrapping the enterostomy with a swab soaked in 1:10,000 topical adrenaline.

Frank bleeding. The blood runs down the abdominal wall and comes usually from a 'pumping' small mesenteric artery deep to the muco-cutaneous junction.

Remove the stitches in that area, lift the mucosa, secure the vessel with fine forceps, and ligate or diathermise.

Luminal bleeding. This is rare and can be mistaken for a muco-cutaneous haemorrhage. It occurs in colostomies when the stools start to become firm, and is secondary to a missed polyp.

144

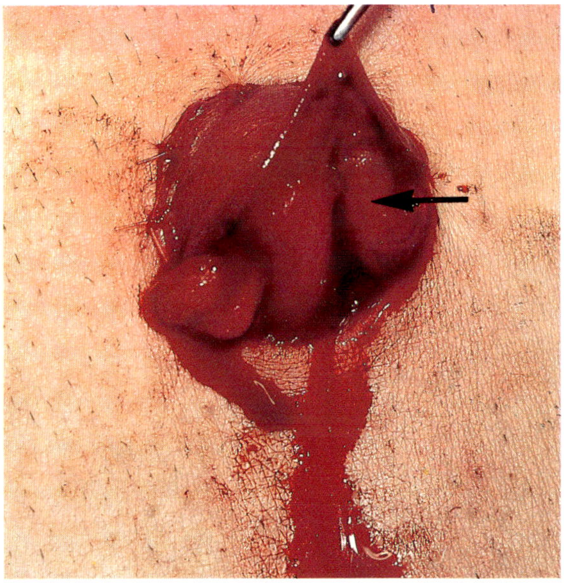

144 Bleeding from a mesenteric vessel (arrowed) within the first 24 post-operative hours. It was fairly brisk, and clots appeared in the pouch.

145

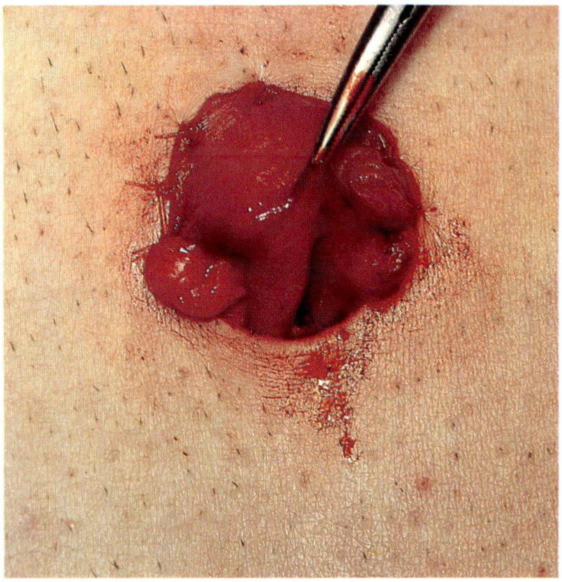

145 *Action required:* Under general anaesthesia or diazepam analepsia unpick the muco-cutaneous sutures. Secure the bleeding point with a haemostat and ligate with catgut. A dry field is obtained the moment the artery has been secured. Replace the muco-cutaneous stitches giving local anaesthesia if diazepam alone has been used.

146

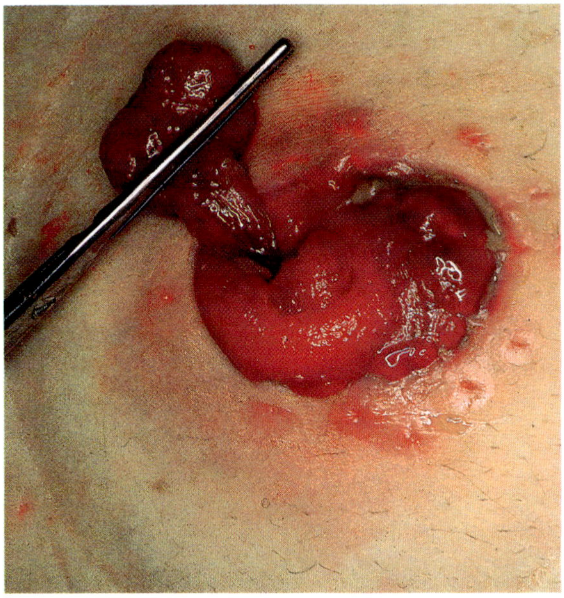

146 An uncommon cause of bleeding from the lumen: a polyp on a stalk.

Action required: Crush the stalk flush with the mucosa; tie with an unabsorbable suture and excise.

Detachment

Can be partial, presenting early or late; or can be circumferential.

Occurs

- usually in the first post-operative week.
- as a complication of retraction.
- in the ill-nourished patient, mostly in association with Crohn's disease.
- from too tight an appliance causing separation or ulceration at the muco-cutaneous junction. This can occur at any time if incorrect size appliance is used.
- secondary to a small subcutaneous or submuccosal abscess or haemorrhage – usually after the first post-operative week, by which time the sutures have dissolved or have been removed.

Management

- when minor, allow to settle. Clean once or twice daily with saline or peroxide, and fill cavity with karaya powder before fixing appliance.
- when major, if retraction is minimal, allow to granulate.
- when major, with marked retraction and the formation of a 'moat' between mucosa and skin, will need refixation or refashioning.

147

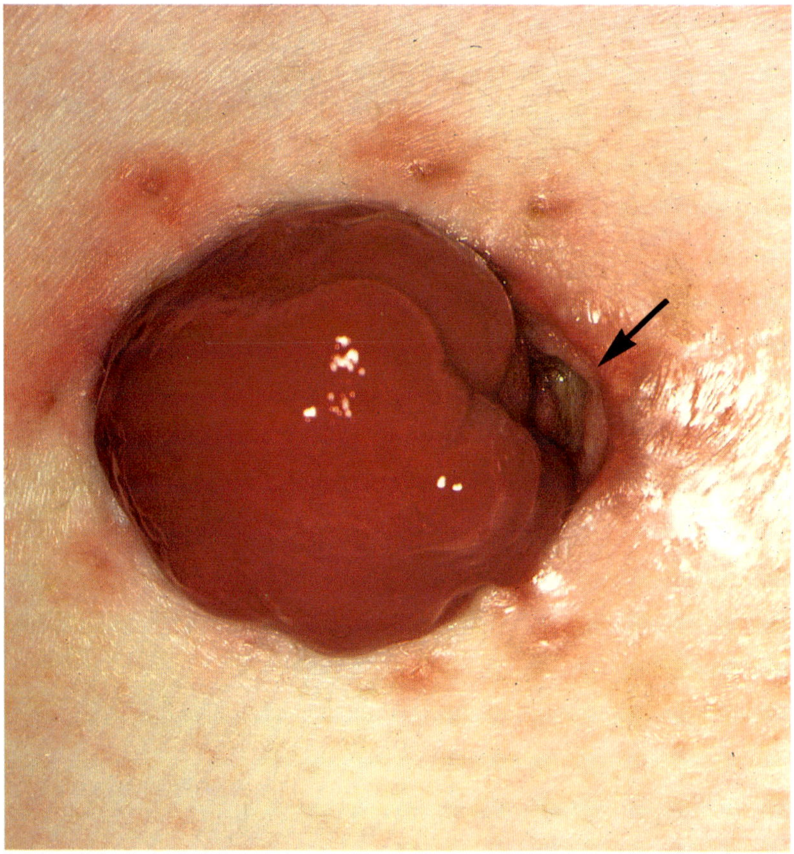

147 A small subcutaneous abscess (arrowed) at 3 o'clock has broken out through the mucosa, a rim of which still remains attached to the skin. Some distortion of the stomal bud has resulted (2nd post operative week).

Action required: Clean daily with saline. Fill cavity with karaya powder before applying a protective wafer, thus allowing granulation to proceed undisturbed.

148

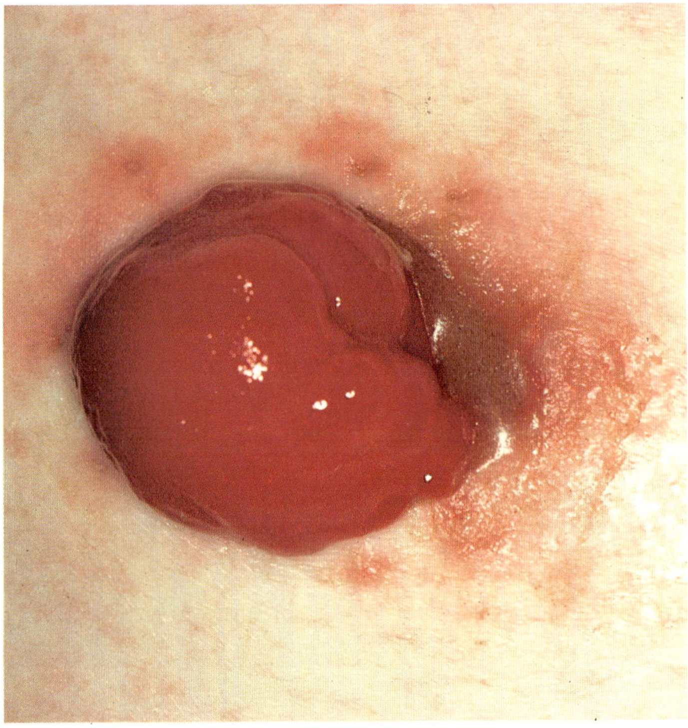

148 The same, with the cavity filled with karaya powder and smoothed down, before applying protective wafer.

149

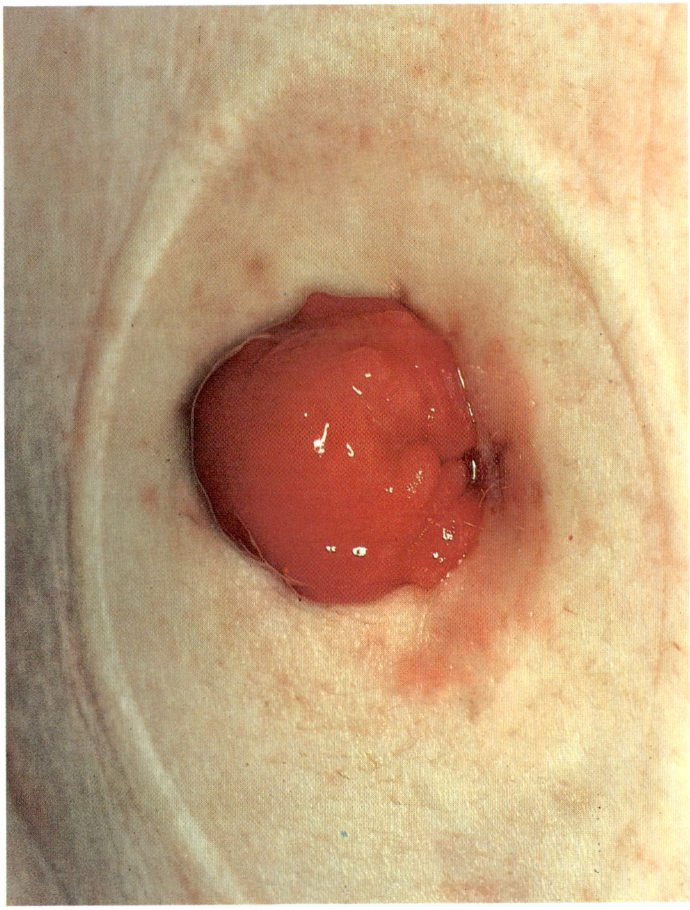

149 The same, four weeks later. There is almost complete healing with minimal distortion of the stoma bud. The appliance fits well, and the peristomal skin is healthy. The stomal bud is still oedematous. Allow it to settle as, once 'mature', the lumen will assume a more central position.

150

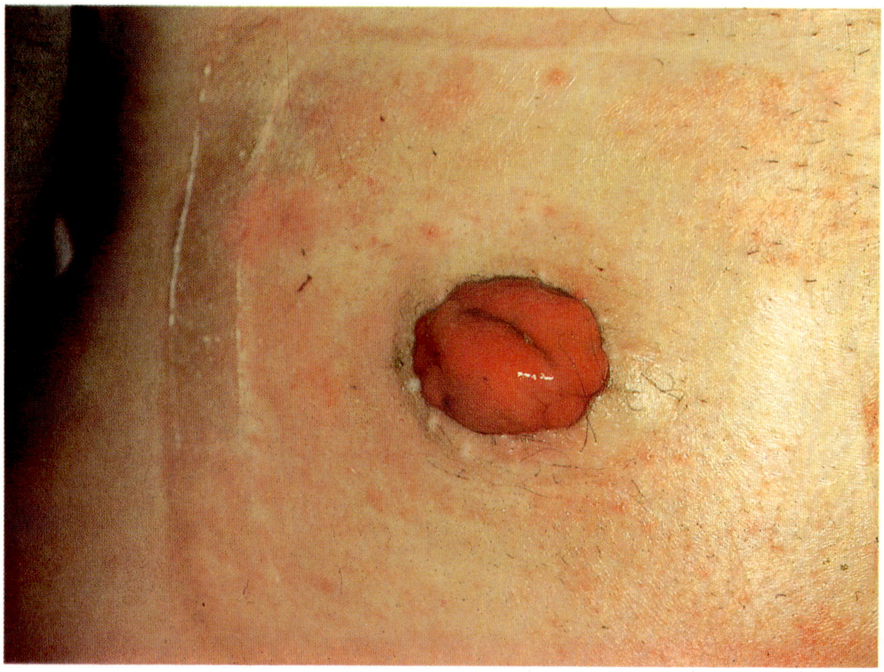

150 Four months later the stoma is almost perfect. The mucosa at the site of the detachment is still irregular and will take several more months to acquire a smooth surface.

151 Too tight an appliance has caused detachment and ulceration (arrowed) in one quadrant, with granulomata in the opposite one.

Action required: Treat detachment as **147**.

151

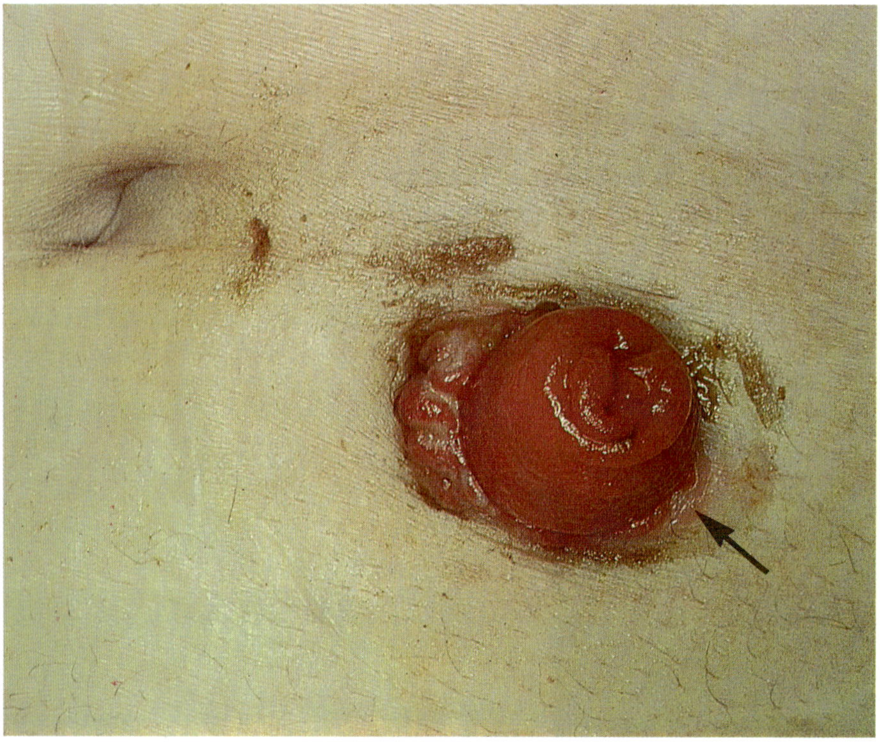

Fistulae

Superficial fistulae usually enter the stoma in that portion of the spout above the muco-cutaneous line. They are usually caused by an unabsorbable suture transfixing the bowel lumen, an event which is followed by infection and a foreign body reaction. They occur early after surgery.

Local necrosis from compression by a rigid appliance can cause a late fistula, especially when the appliance is worn with a belt that pulls upward and damages the inferior border of the stoma.

Spontaneous healing is rare, especially in an ileostomy where the enzyme content of the effluent will digest the tract, interfere with the appliance and keep up the inflammatory process. Nevertheless conservative treatment is worth a trial.

Treatment

Treat with a granulating solution. If unsuccessful, lay the fistula open and allow it to granulate. If this fails, unpick the stoma and refashion it, excluding the fistula. Relocation is rarely necessary.

Deep fistulae occur proximal to the muco-cutaneous level. They result from a peritoneal or fascial suture transfixing the gut deeper than its sero-muscular layer. They present in the early post-operative period. Late fistulae are secondary to an inflammatory process, either in a diverticulum included in the stoma, or in Crohn's disease.

Treatment

Probe the tract; open it up by incising through all layers; remove all fibrous tissue by wide wedge excision down to the serosa. Reconstruct the stoma after amputating the portion beyond the fistula, and suture the wedge, carefully obliterating all dead spaces. A shorter but manageable stoma may result. Follow up for at least a year, as late fibrosis with retraction may occur.

If reconstruction at the same site is not possible, relocate the stoma.

If too flush a stoma is produced in an ileostomy as the result of reconstruction, laparotomy with mobilisation of the ileum may be necessary.

When due to Crohn's disease, the affected bowel must be resected. This requires laparotomy and mobilisation.

152

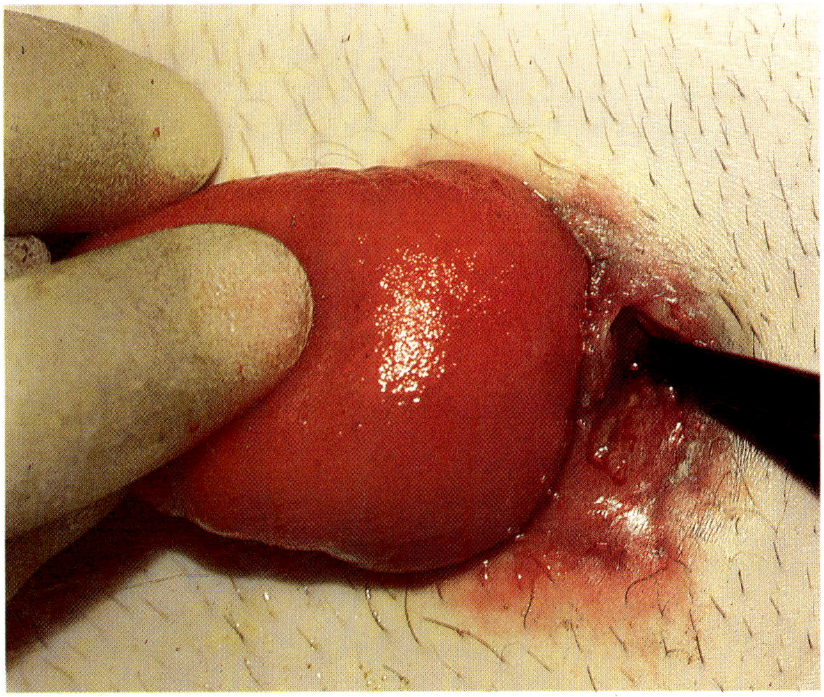

152 A fistula caused by an abscess secondary to an unabsorbable suture at the level of the posterior rectus sheath. Too deep a 'bite' had been taken on the bowel side. With a finger inside the ileostomy, the tip of the probe could be felt just within the trephine hole.

Note the crater formed by digestion of the skin and subcutaneous tissues at the exit site of the fistula.

153

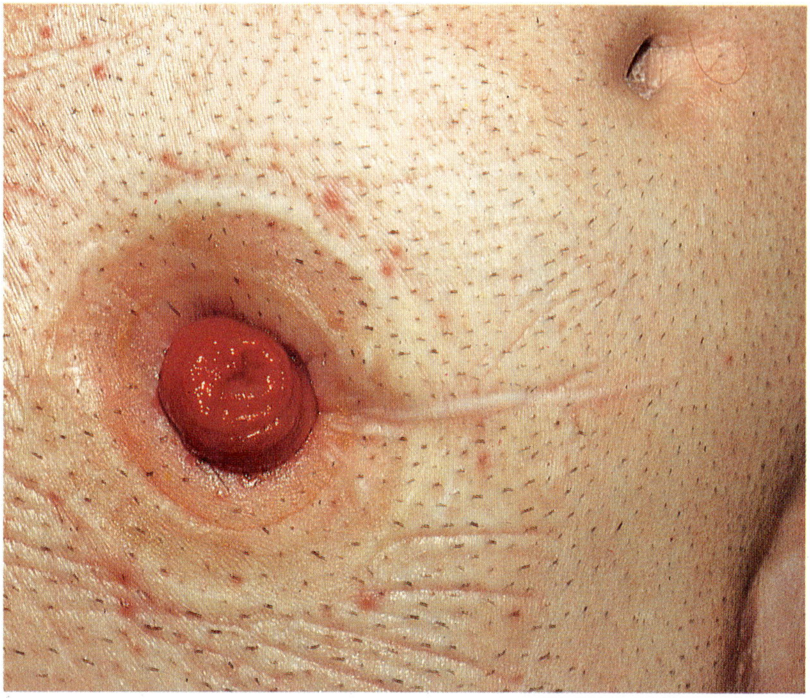

153 A local approach was chosen as the patient was still debilitated from his ulcerative colitis: the fistula was exposed through an incision medial to the ileostomy, which was refashioned. An acceptable result was obtained, with healing by first intention.

154

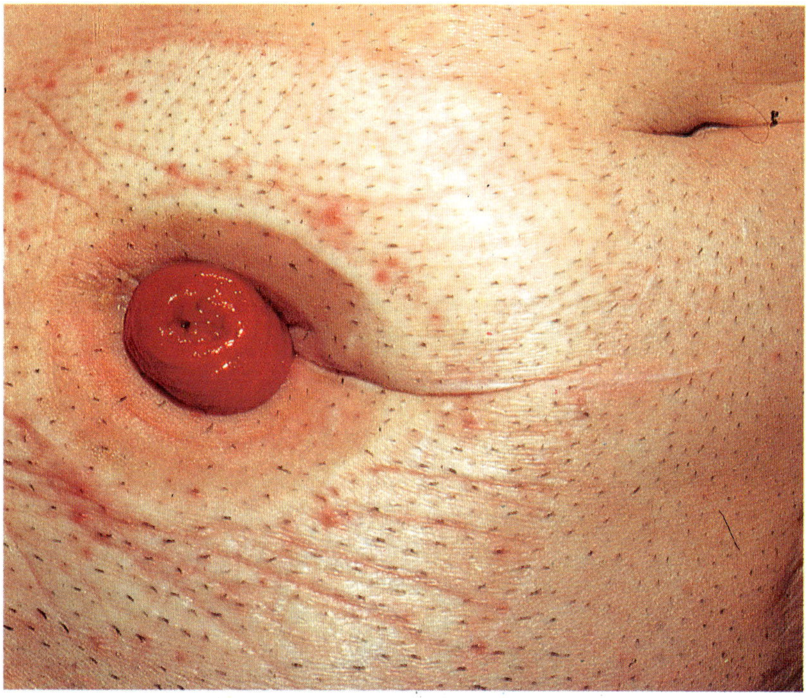

154 Nine months later, the combination of deep-seated fibrosis and substantial weight gain by the patient led to a shelf of skin overhanging the superior aspect of the ileostomy, and 'moat' formation from retraction. Both the shelf and the retraction interfered with the proper fitting of an appliance, causing frequent leaking.

155

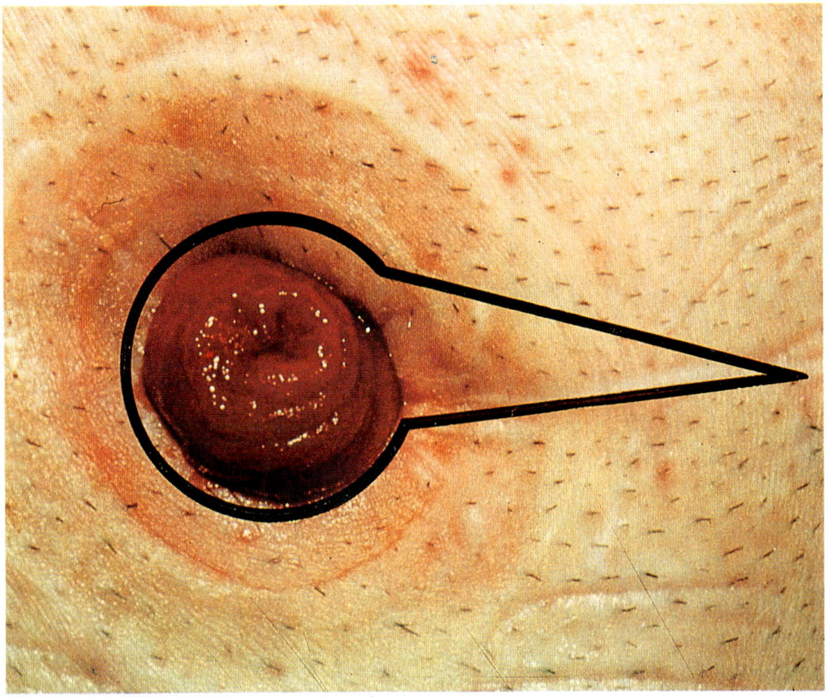

155 The shelf and the fibrous tissue were excised together with excess skin in the fashion marked out on the patient. Fresh skin and subcutaneous fat were rotated to fill in the gap and to fit snugly round the stoma.

156

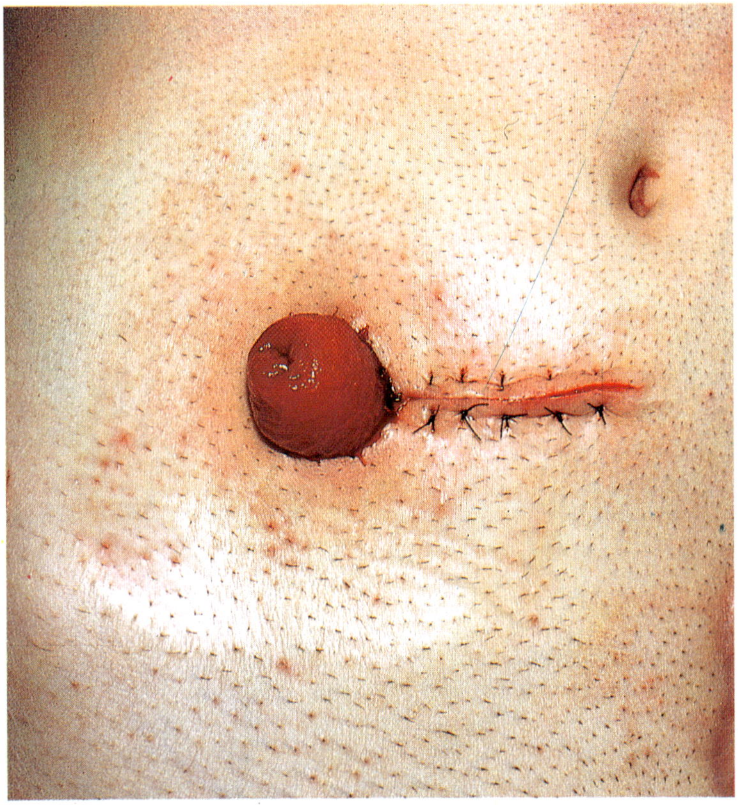

156 A levelled area now surrounds the stoma with disappearance of the shelf and the fibrotic 'moat' deep to the shelf.

157

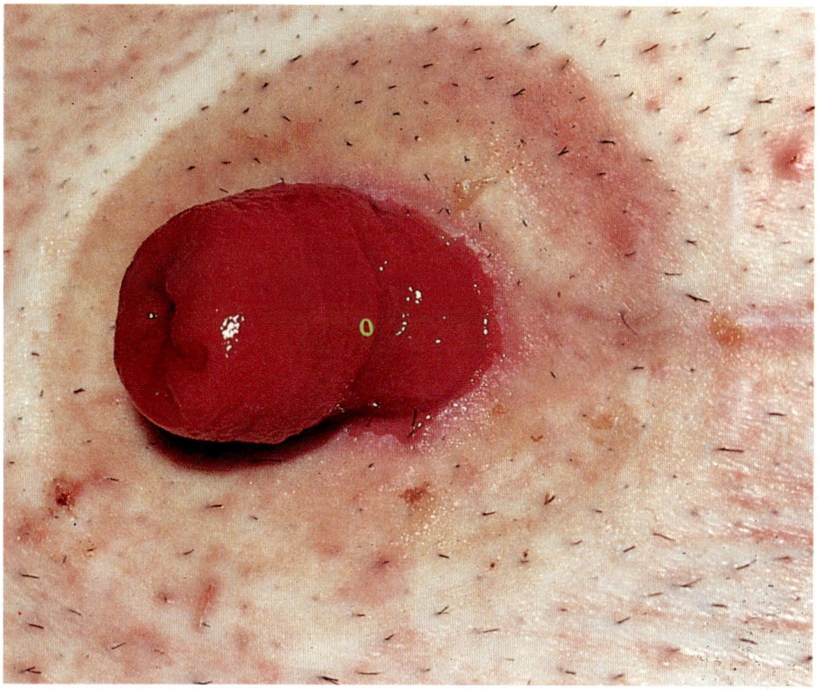

157 The same patient five months later. The stoma is viewed from its medial aspect to show the disappearance of the moat and a better projection of the spout. The well healed medial incision is hardly visible and never interfered with the appliance.

Stenosis

Stenoses can occur early or late. They usually occur at the muco-cutaneous junction, but can occasionally be apical. Since the introduction of the eversion technique they are uncommon.

A stenosis can result from:

- *Poor siting of the stoma,* as in a laparotomy scar, or from too small an excision of a disc of skin, or its construction in a linear incision.
- *Retraction* giving rise to a circumferential inflammatory reaction at the muco-cutaneous junction and the formation of a granulating ring. This leads to the deposition of fibrous or scar tissue which will contract on maturing, producing a rigid stenosis.
- *Ischaemic problems,* either within the stoma itself or at the muco-cutaneous junction. This is more often seen in obese patients with thick mesenteries if too great a length of bowel has been 'skeletonised'.
- *Damage to the apex.* Too long a stoma will impinge against the appliance and be repeatedly bruised. An apical stenosis will result.
- *Crohn's disease* of the stoma.

Management

(1) Daily gentle dilatation with a gloved index finger avoiding fissuring the mucosa.

(2) Use of stool softeners by colostomy patients if they are producing hard stools.

(3) Excision of a larger disc of skin around the stoma and refashioning of the muco-cutaneous junction.

(4) If apical, shorten the stoma by a superficial amputation and resuture.

158

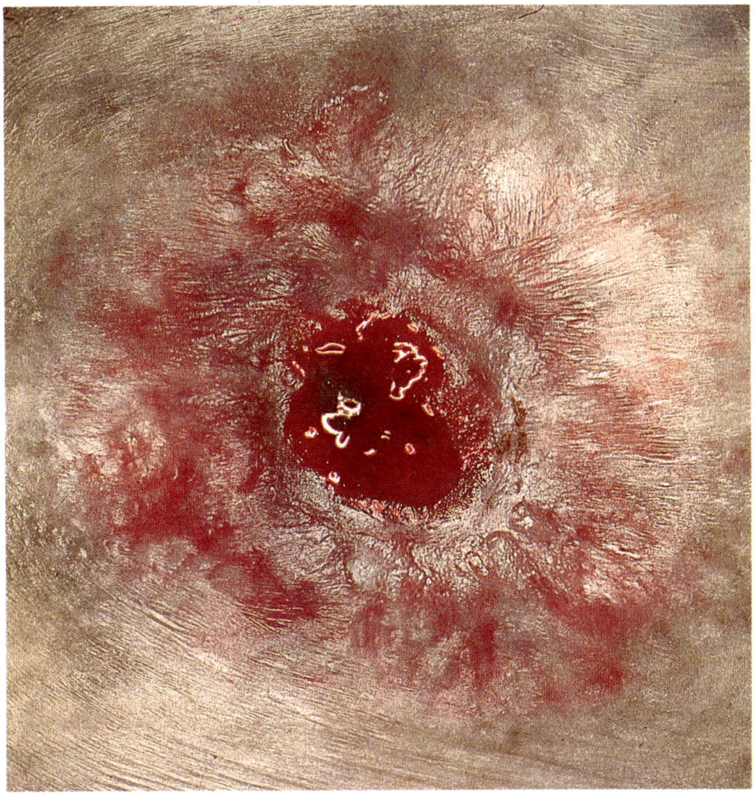

158 Retraction in a colostomy has led to peristomal inflammation of the skin and to scarring of the mucocutaneous junction, lichenification of the skin, and formation of a stenotic ring.

Action required: Actively protect the skin to get it back to a healthy state. Then correct the retraction and refloat the spout.

159

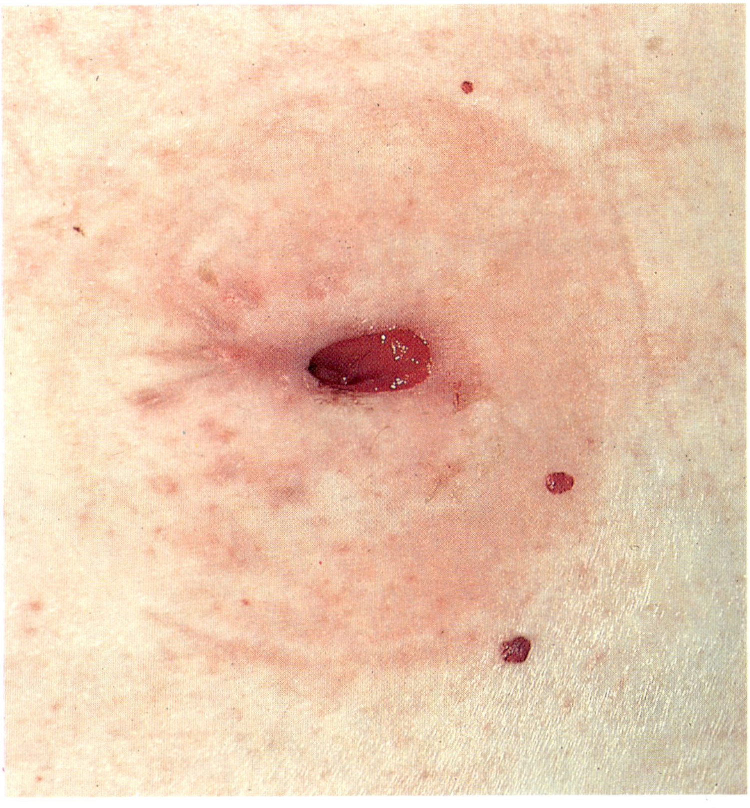

159 A colostomy constructed in a linear incision instead of a trephined hole. Stenosis occurred within weeks of the operation, burying the spout.

Action required: Refashion through a properly trephined hole in the abdominal wall.

160

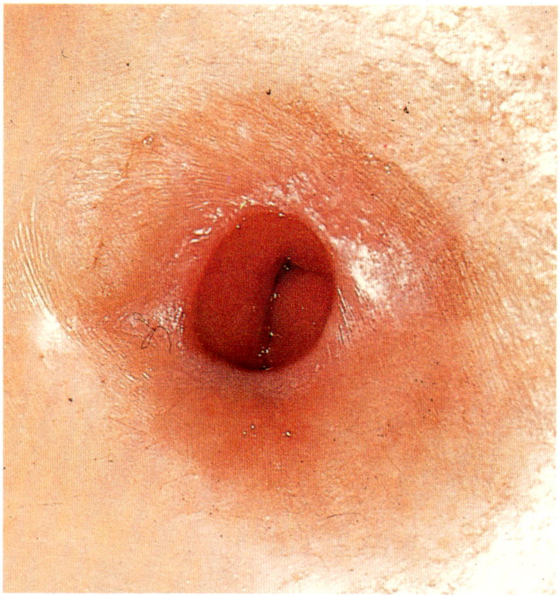

160 The original trephine hole was too small and the spout was too short. Stenosis followed retraction.

161

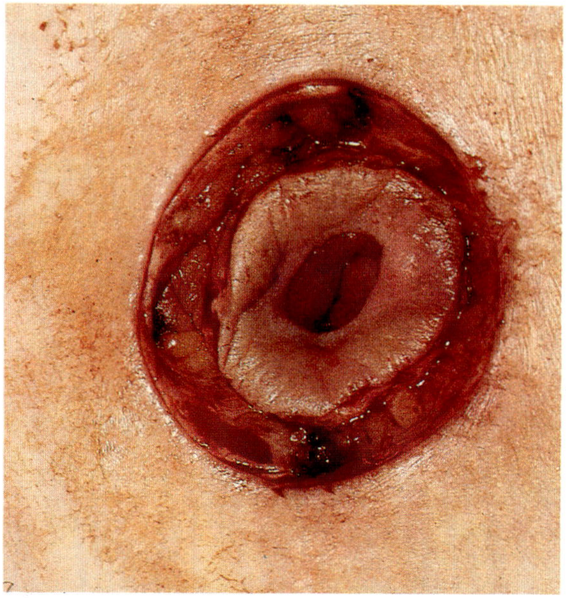

161 Excise a larger circle of skin. Float up the stoma and dissect out the skin 'washer' from the sunken spout. Resuture.

162

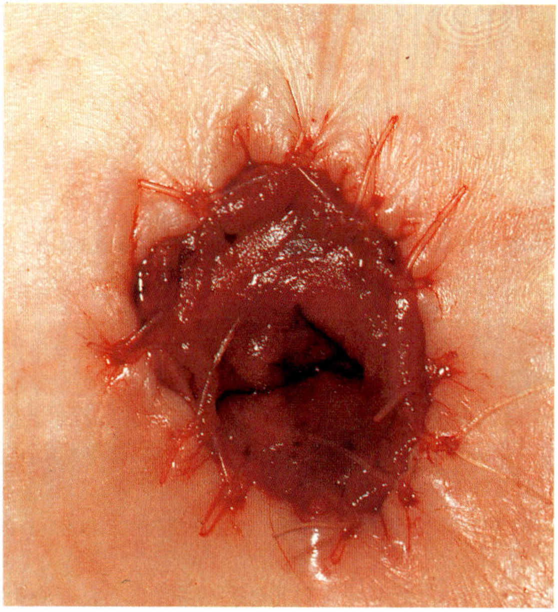

162 Reconstruction of a fresh muco-cutaneous junction to create a good size stoma.

XV: SKIN PROBLEMS

Skin health has more bearing on the patient's well-being than any other factor.

Abdominal skin has a paper-thin horny layer approximately 0.1–0.2 mm thick. Repeated friction or pressure will provoke increased keratinisation, thickening the horny layer for increased protection. Dehydration will make the horny layer crack; excessive hydration, as from increased sweating, leads to maceration. Acute injury causes blisters or vesicles.

Once the macerated epidermis has been breached, the exposed dermis offers no mechanical barrier to infective organisms. Furthermore, proliferation of hair follicles or sweat glands increases the numbers of portals for infection to enter the dermis.

Skin must be dry if an appliance is to adhere properly; equally, loss of natural oils and water will foster skin lesions. This creates a dilemma for the appliance manufacturer, which has been largely resolved since microporous drapes were introduced. Microporosity allows the skin below the adhesive plate to 'breathe', increasing adherence without causing maceration.

Healthy skin has a pH of around 5 and is more vulnerable to damage from alkalis than acids. Intestinal contents can damage it owing to their high pH and enzymes, an effect that is worse from ileostomies and right transverse colostomies than sigmoid colostomies.

Chemical damage and allergic reactions cause rashes.

Contact dermatitis is uncommon with hypo-allergenic adhesives; nevertheless it can be severe when it does occur and requires active treatment.

Minor trauma caused by the adhesive square will cause transient dermatitis in at least 50% of patients. It bothers the patients for only a few days a year and is of little consequence. Patients should be forewarned of its likelihood and, if they report it, reassured of its benign and fleeting nature.

Age and nutritional status play a part in skin health – depleted oil and keratin production, due to advancing age or poor nutrition, are an important factor in stubborn skin problems. Many skin problems can be forestalled by correcting malnutrition preoperatively. Elderly and malnourished people with impaired skin health will benefit from an appliance that does not require frequent changing.

The combination of all the above factors, to which must be added the psychological trauma of an altered self-image, brings about a fairly uniform pattern of skin problems – they are worst in the first two post-operative months, and slowly improve until, by the end of the first year as the skin horny layer thickens beneath the appliance, and the patient regains his or her well-being, they disappear almost totally. By then, patients have settled down to a routine and the use of their definitive appliance.

Only when pre-existing dermatoses are present (e.g. ichthyosis, psoriasis, eczema, etc) is the pattern different and requires the help of an expert dermatologist.

Skin problems

Specific aspects

There are three main groups of peri-stomal dermatitis:

A. Insult dermatitis.
B. Contact dermatitis, which may be chemical or allergic..
C. Infective dermatitis.

Insult dermatitis

This is essentially the result of mechanical trauma to the skin. It can be due to:

(1) Microscopical skin tears from over-vigorous cleaning of the skin round the stoma. Soft soap, warm water and cotton wool are the kindest cleaning agents and should be used in preference to any other.

(2) Blocking of skin pores by the waterproof adhesive square. Maceration results and leads to infection. Microporous adhesive plates have virtually eliminated this problem.

(3) Over-frequent changing of the adherent appliance. The epidermal cells are progressively stripped off, with loss of the protective horny layer.

(4) Incorrect application of the adhesive square. If tension is applied to it during fixing, a shearing effect can result between epidermis and dermis with complete loss of the former on stripping the appliance. Non-stretch adhesive squares have minimised this problem.

Contact dermatitis

Chemical

This is due to the direct irritant or corrosive effect of the chemical on the skin. It will start *immediately* and will be sharply defined.

There is first erythema, then desquamation, followed by a burning sensation typical of physical damage to the skin.

Faecal seepage from an ill-fitting appliance is the commonest cause, its pH and enzyme content affecting the skin. It is at its most prevalent in the early days and must be prevented in the immediate post-operative period by applying a well-fitting adherent drainable bag on the operating table and leaving it on as long as possible. Once the stoma is working, the pouch should be emptied frequently to diminish the duration of exposure of the skin to the effluents.

In the past, zinc oxide plaster was used and zinc could affect the skin directly. Similarly, ether meth, trichlorethane (Zoff) and tincture of benzoin (Friars' Balsam) were in current use and injured the epidermis. Modern adhesives have rendered these obsolete. Detergents and deodorants are harmful chemicals when used over-zealously.

Allergic

This cannot take place without previous exposure to the allergens, and therefore a delay of weeks or years will precede the appearance of the reaction. Itching is common and, though the hypersensitivity is limited to the area of contact with the allergens, the reaction can spread quickly beyond it.

Any element of the appliance can be at fault: rubber, plastic, nickel, chromium, zinc, adhesives, solvents; as can be the effluents, particularly after antibiotic therapy. A careful history often reveals that an antibiotic diarrhoea preceded the condition.

Allergic reactions can severely damage the skin and usher in septic dermatitis. Treatment is by separating all suspect agents from the skin and using topical steroids and even sometimes systemic steroids. However, long-term use of topical steroids can lead to skin atrophy and make matters worse.

Patch testing is recommended preoperatively in anyone with a previous history of allergy, including migraine.

Infective dermatitis

This is almost always grafted on to an insult or a contact dermatitis. The bacterial flora of the gut as well as the skin is altered by constructing a stoma, and may well be an important factor. So are malnutrition and coexisting conditions such as diabetes.

Infection is usually both bacterial and fungal. The former usually staphylococcal and coliform, the latter *Candida* (thrush). Topical antibiotics and antifungals are useful in the treatment of this condition after culture of organisms and sensitivity testing.

Individuals prone to eczema – atopic or seborrhoeic – are more susceptible to infective dermatitis.

XIV: PERISTOMAL SKIN

163

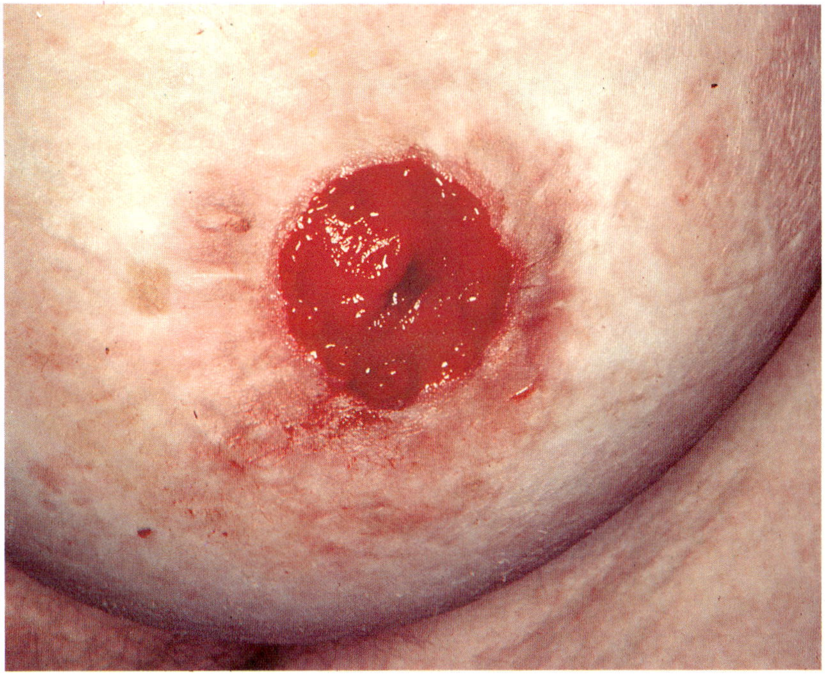

163 Insult dermatitis: early stage. A flush or retracted stoma due to herniation. In the sitting position the face-plate tended to become unstuck. The patient therefore changed the appliance frequently. Early damage to the skin ensued, visible as tiny tears with ecchymoses and sanguineous blisters.

Action required: Apply the pouch in the sitting position using, if necessary, a two-piece appliance held by a belt until the skin has healed. If it is not controlled by conservative means the hernia may need to be corrected surgically. Note the pyogenic granulomata in the stomal mucosa.

164

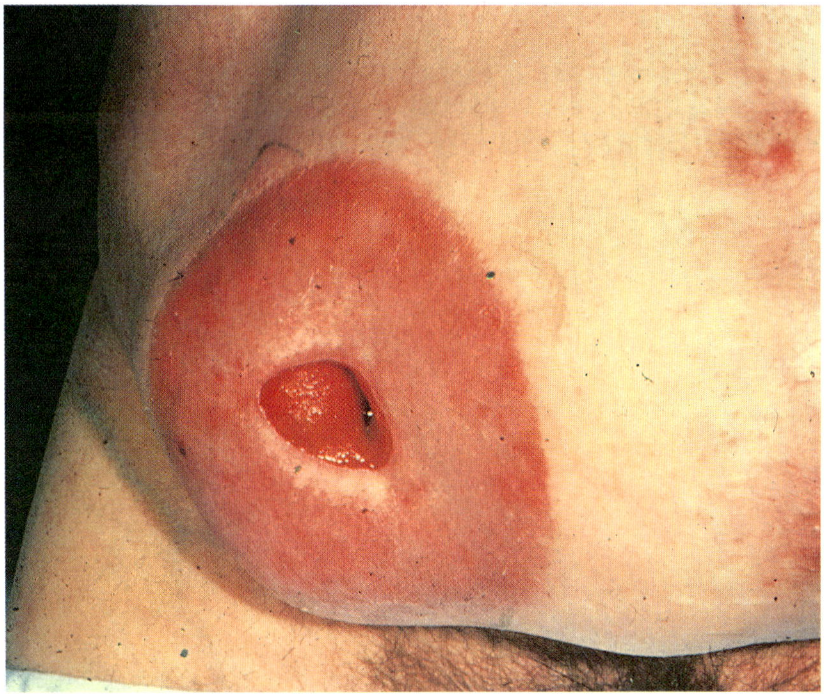

164 Insult dermatitis: late stage. Frequent changing of the appliance has led to skin damage, further affected by faecal leaking under the plate. The damage is characteristically limited to the area of the face-plate.

Action required: Apply a protective wafer, moulding it as closely as possible to the contours of the herniated bulge. Fix it further with adhesive tape if necessary. The wafer offers a surface on which to stick a pouch and can be left for as long as it remains attached. Failure to heal may require hernial repair or relocation of the stoma.

165
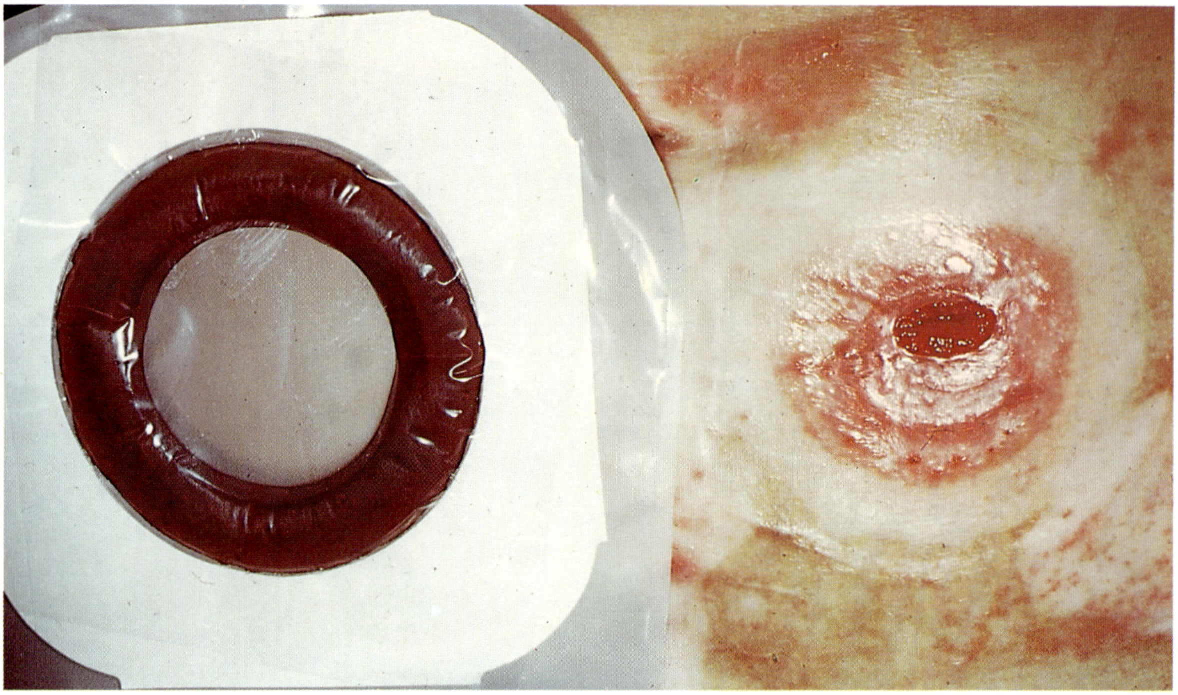

165 Chemical dermatitis. Too wide an appliance is a fairly common cause of peristomal skin damage.

Action required: Change to the correct size appliance. The skin will quickly re-epithialise and all soreness disappear.

166
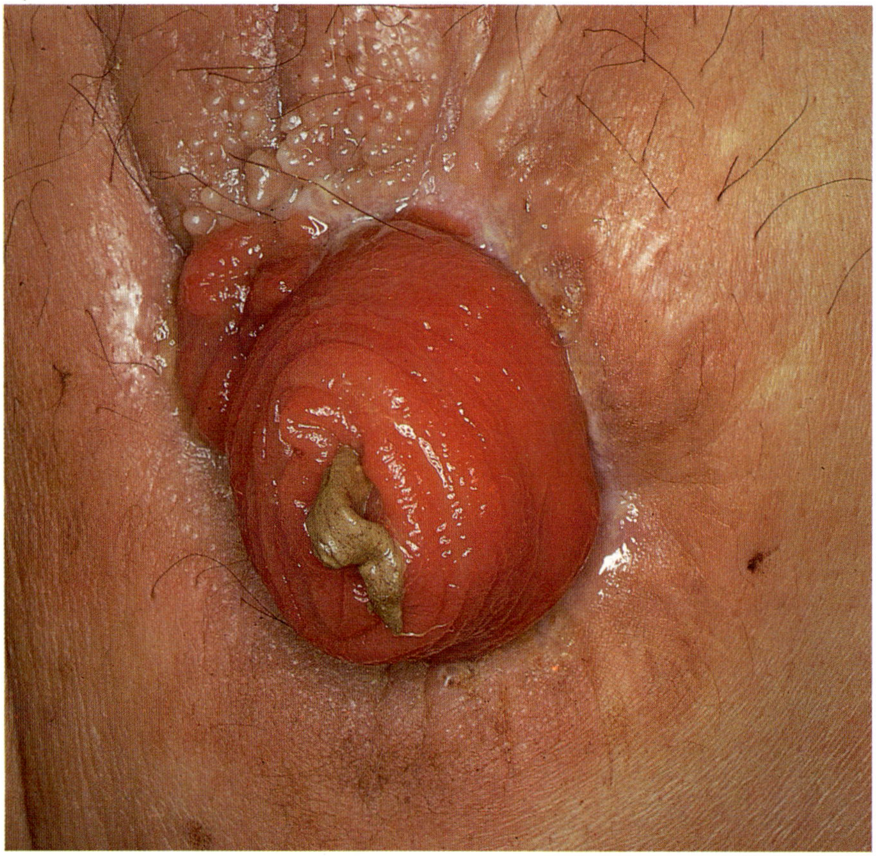

166 Chemical dermatitis. Defunctioning ileostomy in Crohn's disease, following breakdown of an ileocolic anastomosis. Skin maceration by enzymes, with bullae formation; is visible.

Action required: Protect the skin with a karaya, stomahesive or similar wafer. Refashion the anastomosis as soon as possible, and restore ileal continuity once anastomosis is fully healed.

167

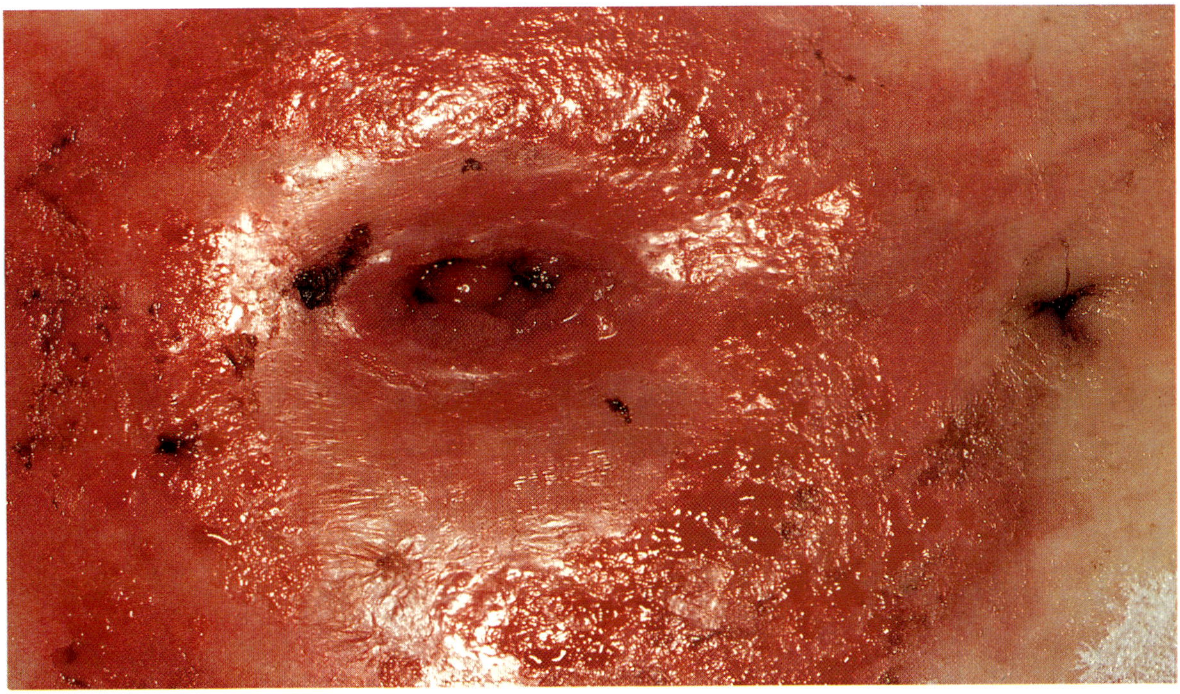

167 Chemical dermatitis. Severe faecal dermatitis around a right transverse colostomy that retracted completely after its supporting rod was removed too early. The enzyme-rich effluent has burnt and blistered the skin, which bled superficially each time an appliance was changed.

Action required: Protect the skin as much as possible to minimise the contact dermatitis. Closure or refashioning of the colostomy is the only lasting solution to such a problem.

168

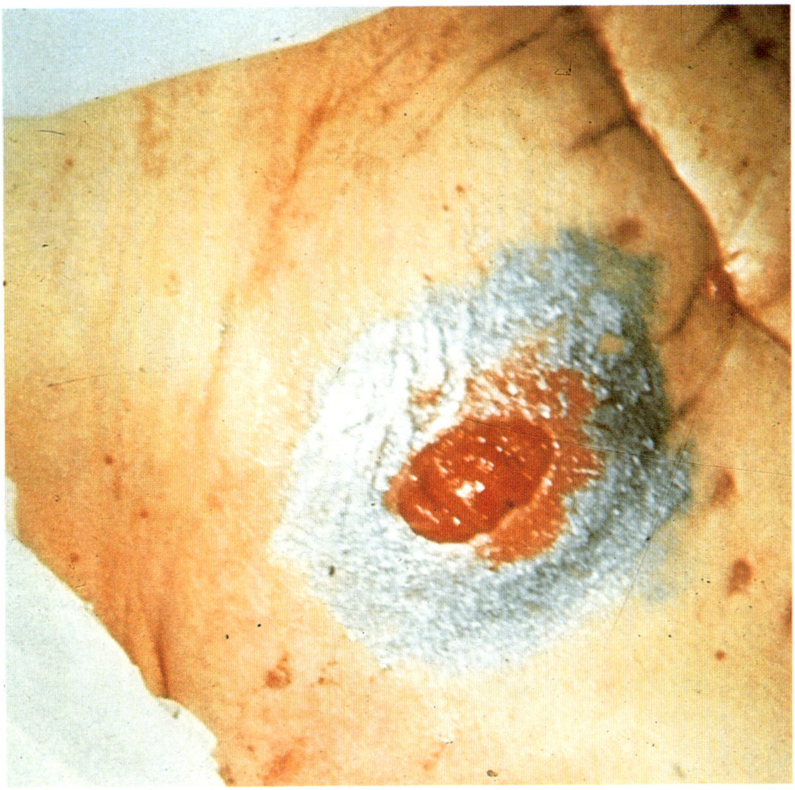

168 'Ballerina paste' was a major standby for skin protection against faecal dermatitis in the early days of stoma care. It has been superseded by most of the modern barrier creams and protective wafers, but has still many advocates.

169

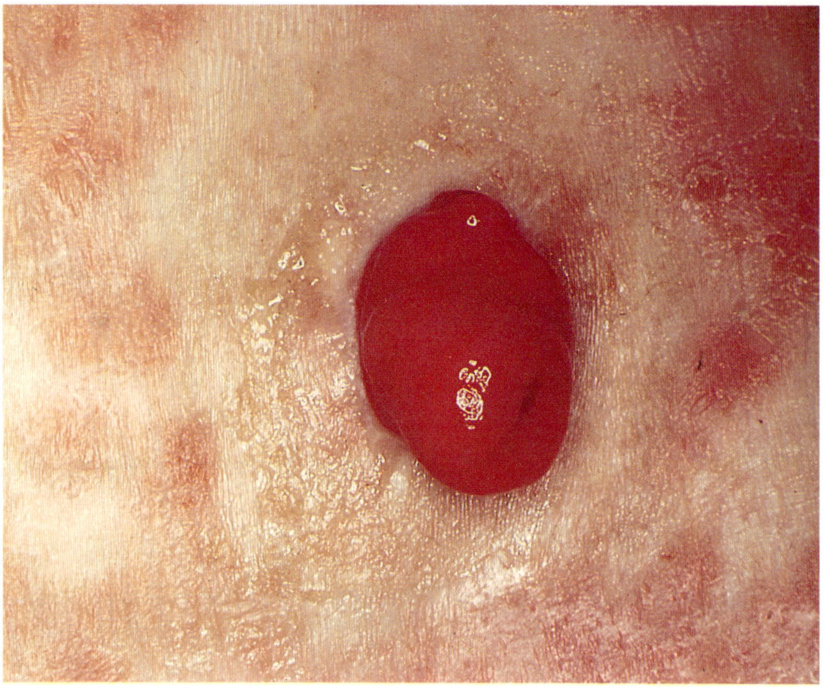

169 *Contact dermatitis* (allergic). Early contact dermatitis from the adhesive of the backing plate. Small pustules are present from superadded infection.

Action required: Change the appliance using one with a protective wafer if necessary. Steroid impregnated tape (see appendix) can be very helpful in such a condition. The tape is applied across the affected areas, and the appliance adheres to the tape.

170

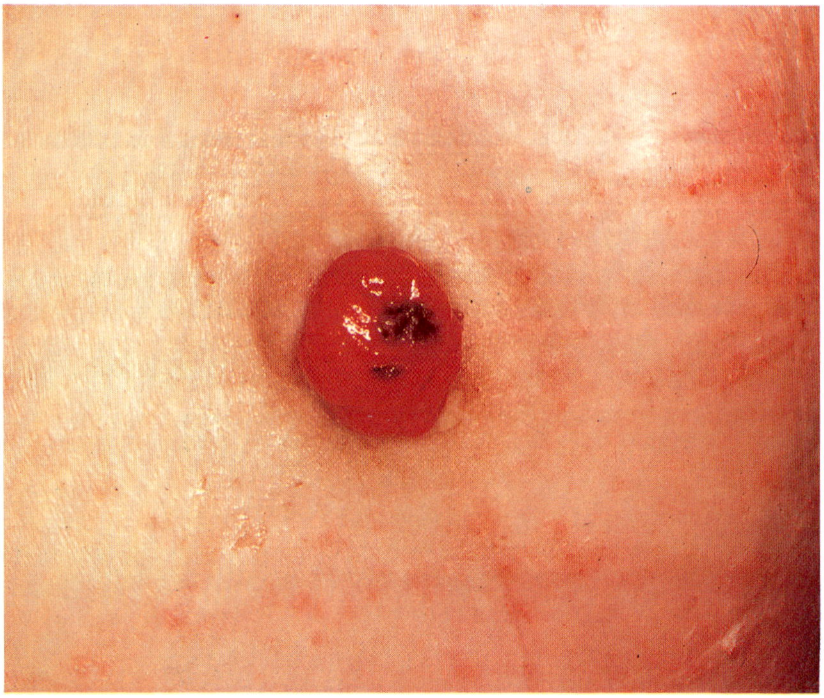

170 The same patient four weeks after the use of a steroid tape. The allergic reaction has been controlled and the skin is almost back to normal. Steroid preparations when correctly used are invaluable and give rewarding results.

171

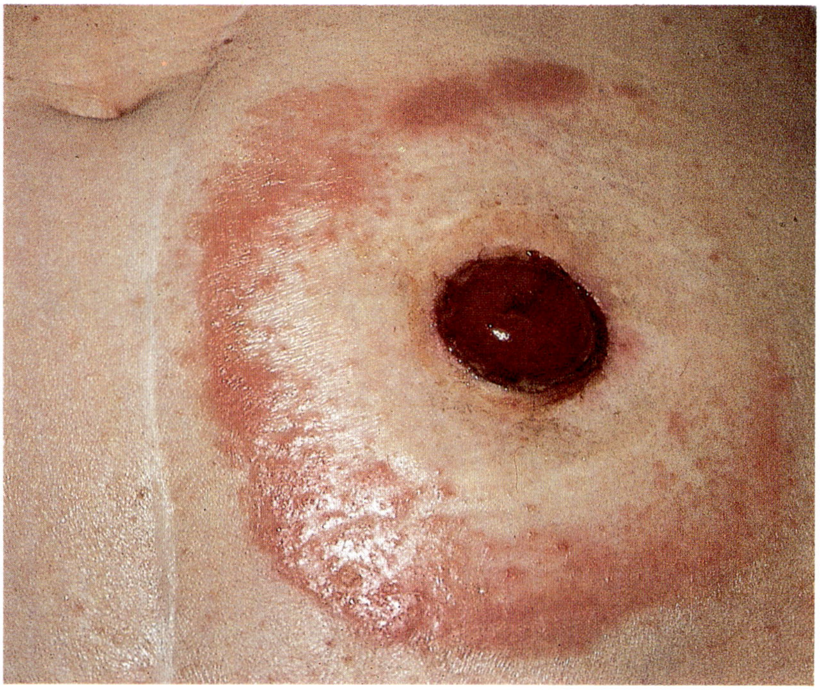

171 *Contact dermatitis* (allergic). A similar, but more severe adhesive contact dermatitis than that shown in **169** with the reaction spreading beyond the area of contact – even underneath the karaya gum ring. (It should be remembered that some patients may develop a sensitivity to Karaya itself.)

Action required: Replace the appliance, preferably with one without an adhesive and backed just with a protective wafer. Treat the affected area with a steroid impregnated tape.

172

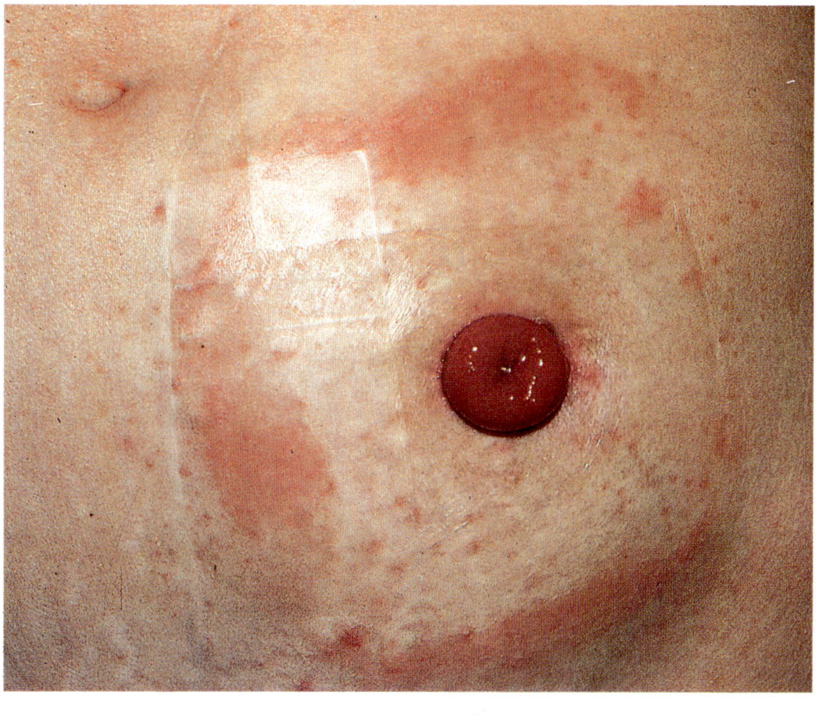

172 The same patient one week later, with some strips of the tape left *in situ*. A good response has been obtained, the dermatitis fading rapidly with spontaneous remission of the surface infection.

173

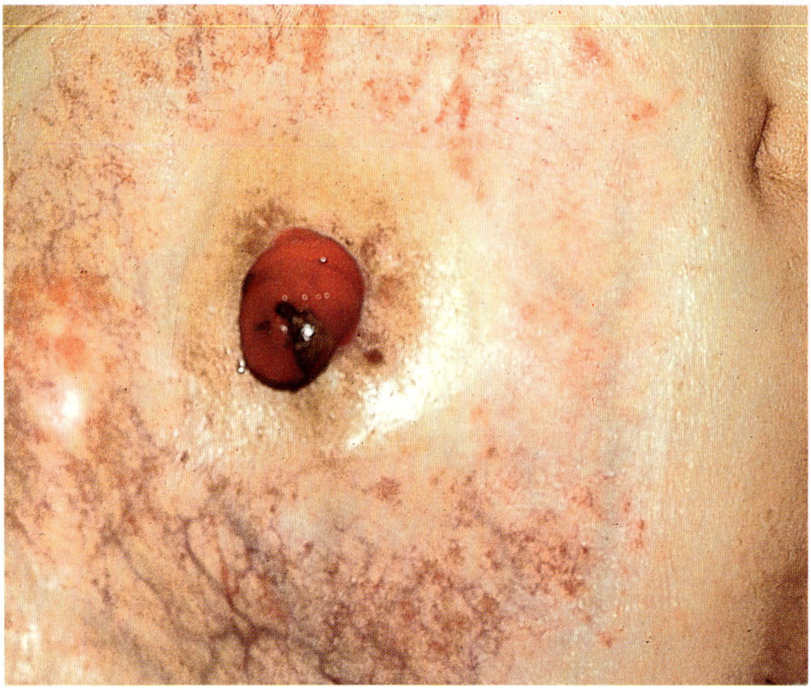

173 Unfortunately the patient suffered further episodes of contact dermatitis with other appliances, failed to keep her follow-up appointments and went on treating herself with the steroid releasing tape. Three years later she reported with a paper thin transparent skin typical of steroid misuse. Discontinuance of the use of the tape resulted in partial skin recovery.

174

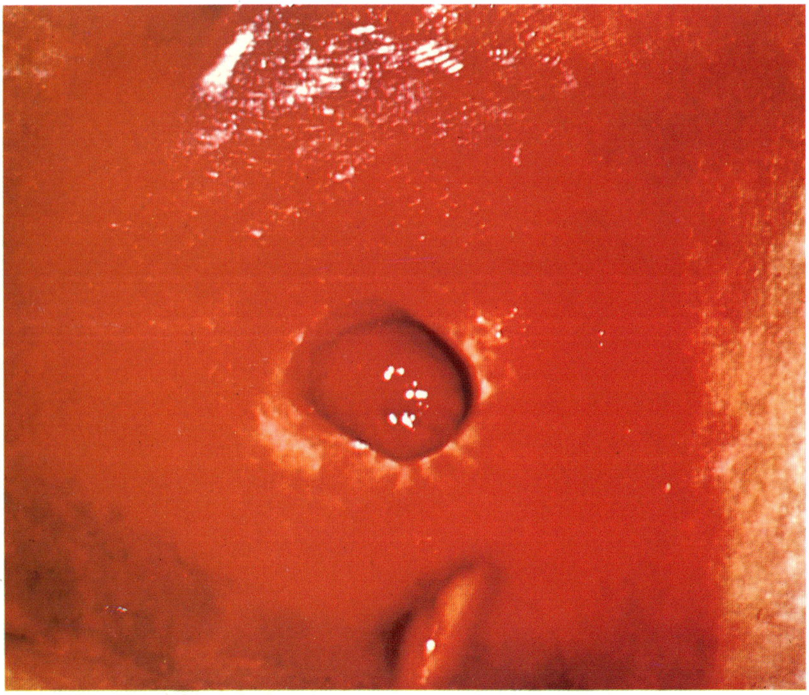

174 A severe case of dermatitis with multiple causes. A florid allergic reaction a few weeks after operation led to detachment of the ileostomy, with a chemical dermatitis complicating the picture. A staphylococcal infection rapidly supervened to produce the haemorrhagic state shown. The patient was hypoproteinaemic.

Action required: Correct the nutritional state, preferably parenterally using a high calorie high protein regimen. Enteral feeding, if used, should be of a low or no-residue variety. Give the appropriate systemic antibiotic. Protect the skin in every possible manner until the patient is fit enough for refashioning or relocating of the ileostomy. A defunctioning ileostomy has a place here.

XVII: THE SKIN UNDER THE POUCH

175

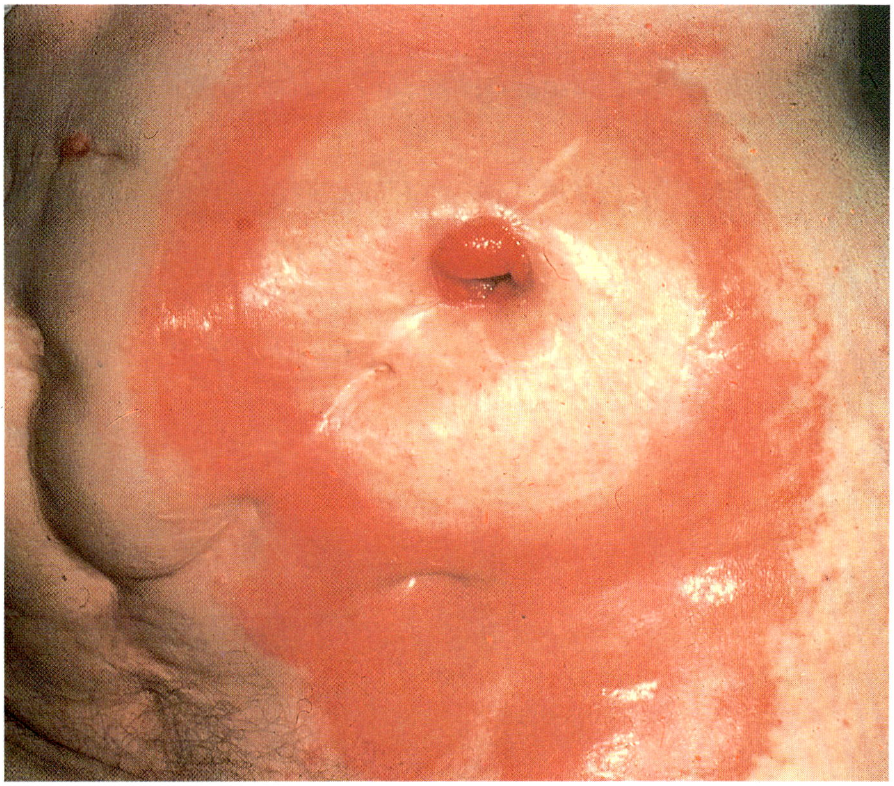

75 Allergic dermatitis. Over a year after starting using a plastic pouch, the patient reacted to it. The skin under the circular wafer suffered no contact and remained unaffected.

Action required: Change the make of the pouch. The use of hypo-allergic material has virtually eliminated this problem.

176

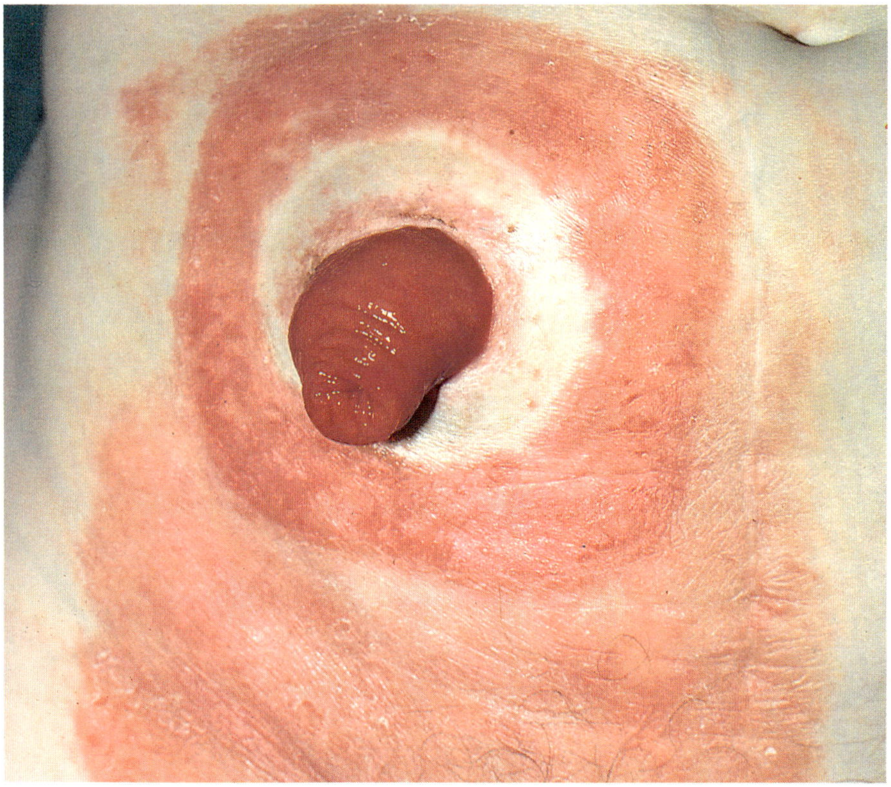

176 Allergic dermatitis. Reaction to the adhesive of the face plate. The area underneath the incorporated protective wafer is not affected. Note that the reaction has spread beyond the area of the face plate and has invaded the perimeter of the protective wafer. A milder reaction to the pouch itself is also present.

Action required: Use an appliance of a different make, with a larger protective wafer. Apply a steroid cream if necessary.

XVIII: THE PERI-INTESTINAL AREA

The main peri-intestinal condition is herniation, which is commoner in ileostomies than colostomies. Intestinal loops escape through the abdominal wall alongside the stoma. A sac forms between layers of subcutaneous fascial planes, often not obliterated during construction of the stoma.

Herniation lateral or medial to the stoma separates the cut edges of the rectus muscle and creates a neck that tends to be linear in shape.

Herniation above or below the stoma displaces the cut edge of the rectus upwards or downwards, forming a defect which is semicircular and not always easy to repair.

The general policy is to overcome the problem by transplanting the stoma. However, careful and accurate repair of the defect using the standard principles of corrective surgery can be highly successful and will avoid the major problems of translocation.

177

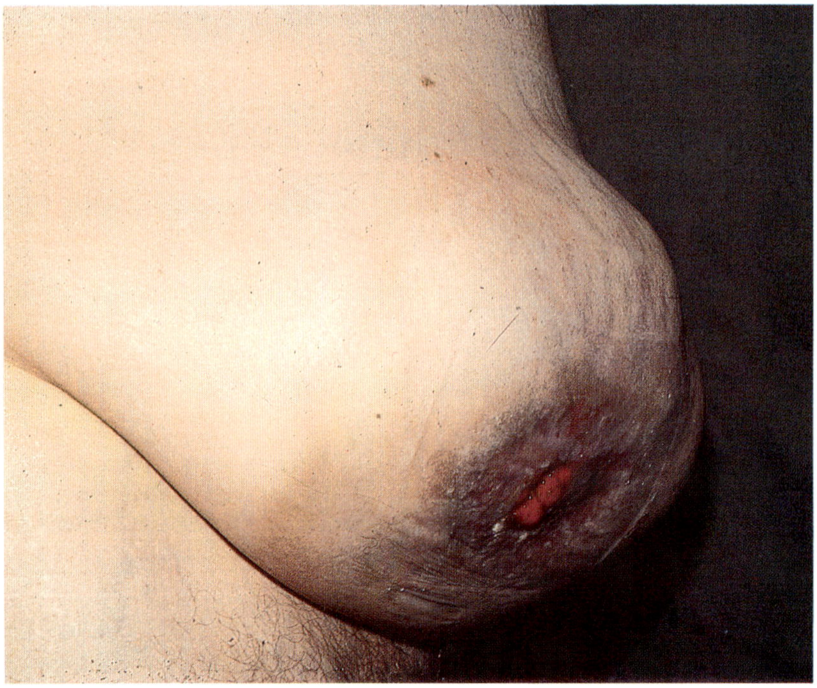

177 Gross herniation of an ileostomy in a patient who had gained 15 kg in the two years since surgery. The stoma has retracted and the small bowel had herniated through a linear defect lateral to the ileostomy and lay in a large circumferential pendulous subcutaneous sac. Appliances were difficult to fit and skin damage was a recurring problem.

178

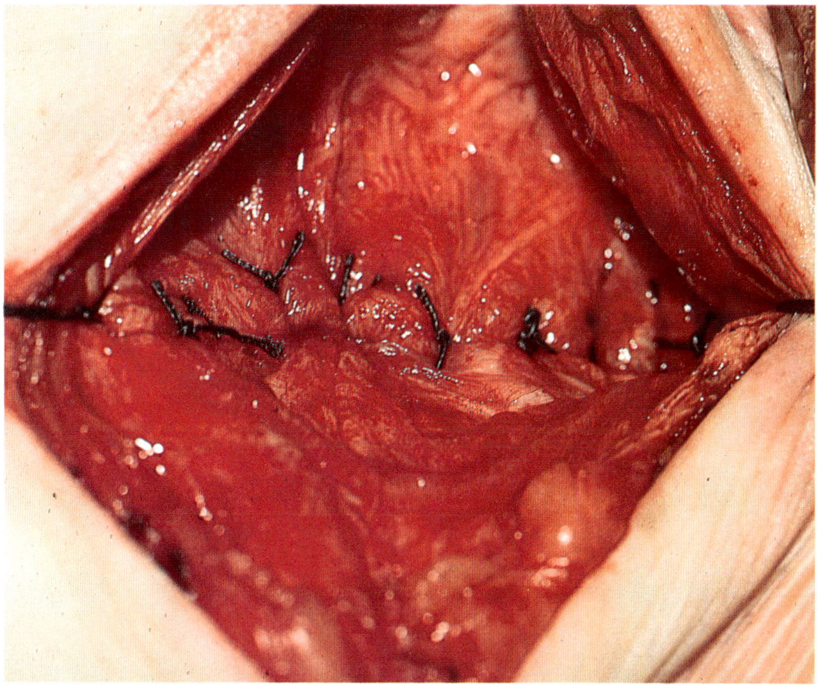

178 Via a horizontal incision lateral to the stoma, the sac was exposed, its contents were reduced and it was excised. The muscular defect was repaired in layers using unabsorbable sutures.

179

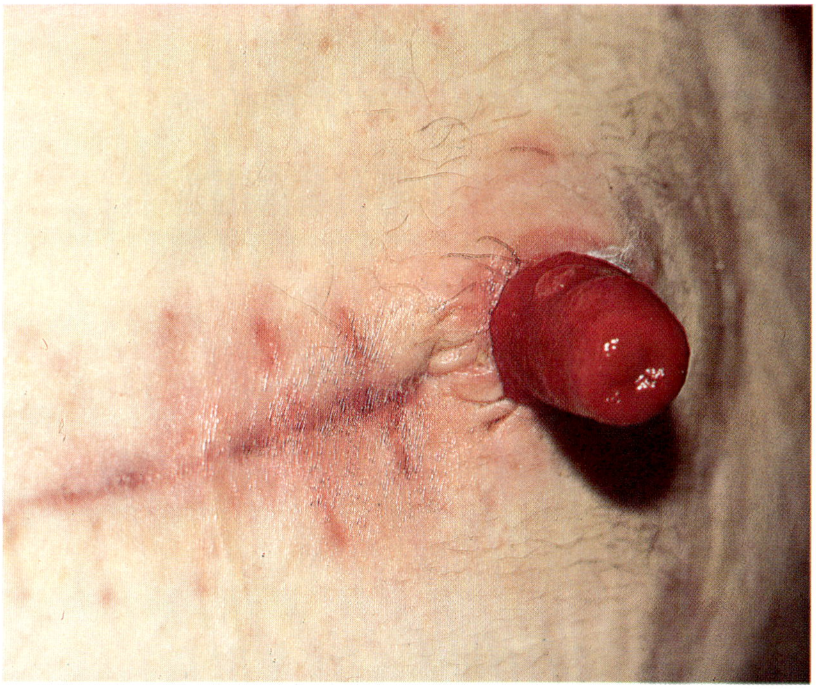

179 The result four weeks after surgery. The stomal spout has re-exteriorised itself without the need for any refashioning.

180

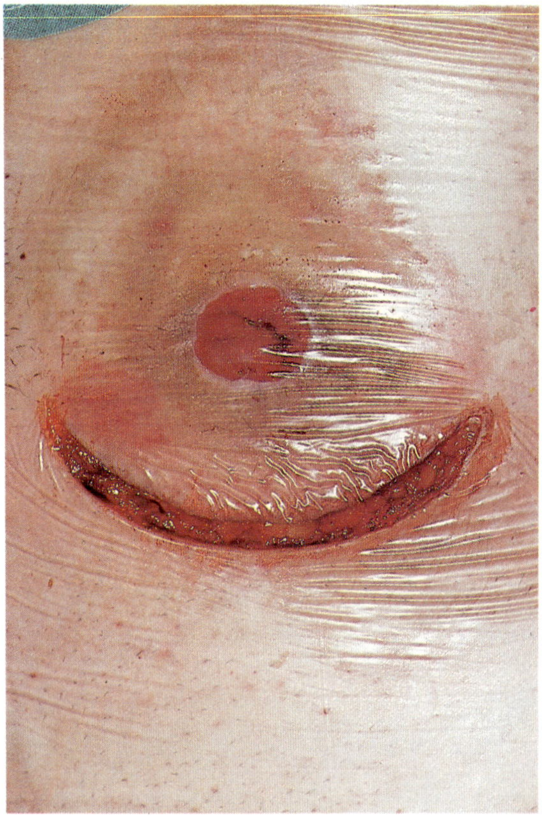

180 A substomal herniation leading to retraction. A curved incision is made below the inferior limits of the sac down to the anterior rectus sheath, through the full thickness of the subcutaneous fatty layers.

181

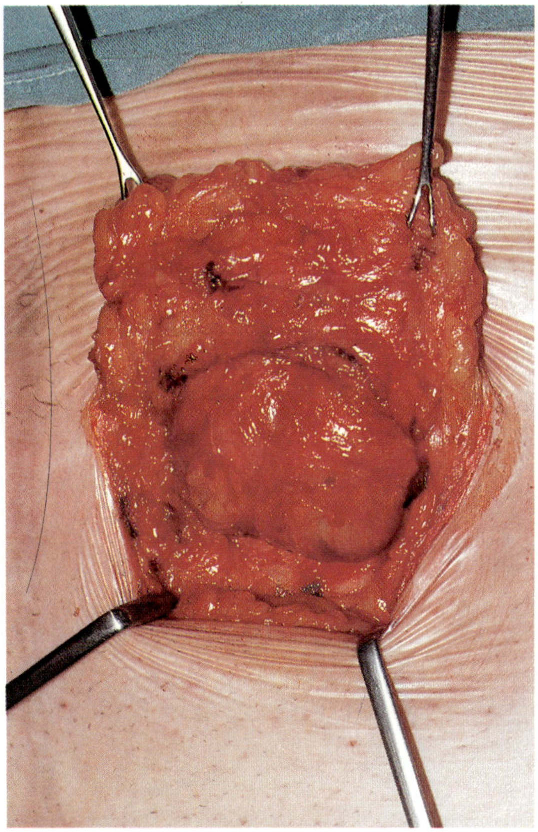

181 Skin and subcutaneous fat are lifted *en bloc* from the sac right up to the level of the stoma.

182
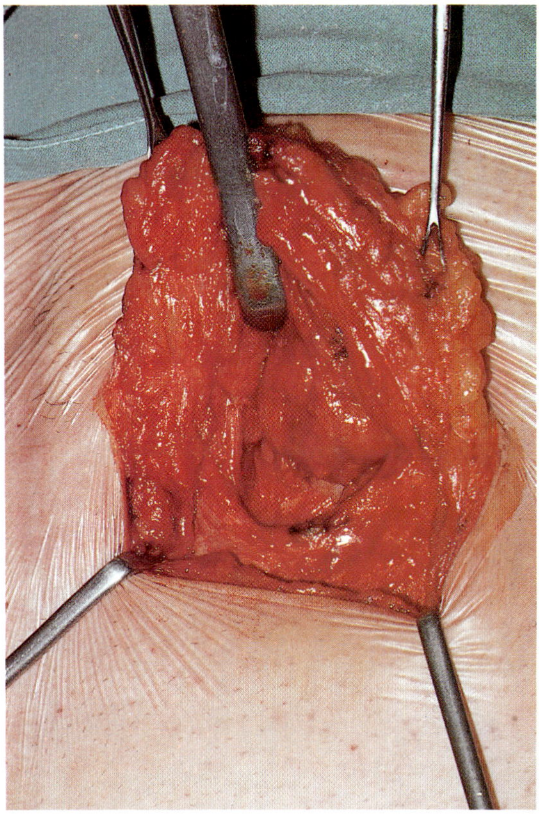

182 The sac is dissected cleanly from the rectus sheath and muscle to expose the sharp edges of the neck of the sac.

183
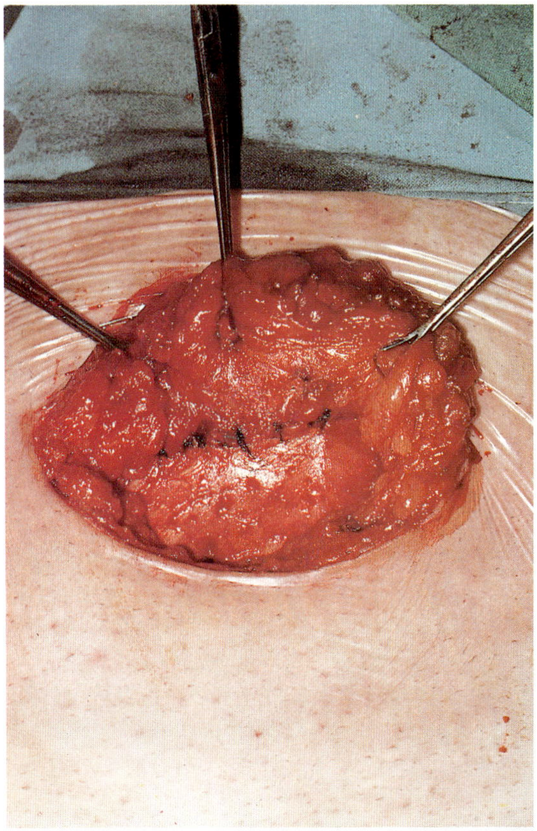

183 After dissecting the respective planes of the rectus muscle and reducing the sac, repair is undertaken in layers using unabsorbable sutures. The skin and its subcutaneous layers of fat are then carefully resutured. Exacting haemostasis is mandatory.

184

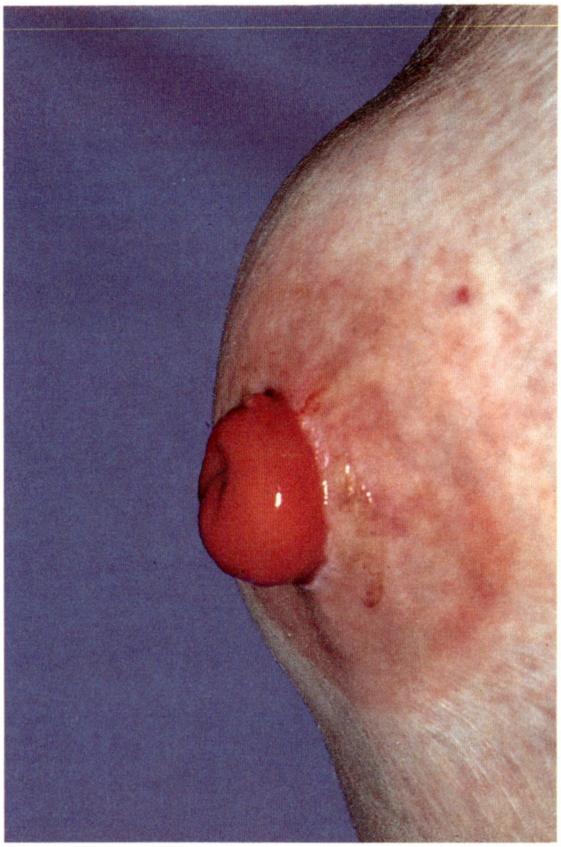

184 A supra-stomal hernia in a colostomy. When standing, the bulge prevented the appliance fitting properly. The skin is thinning out and is becoming prone to injury.

185

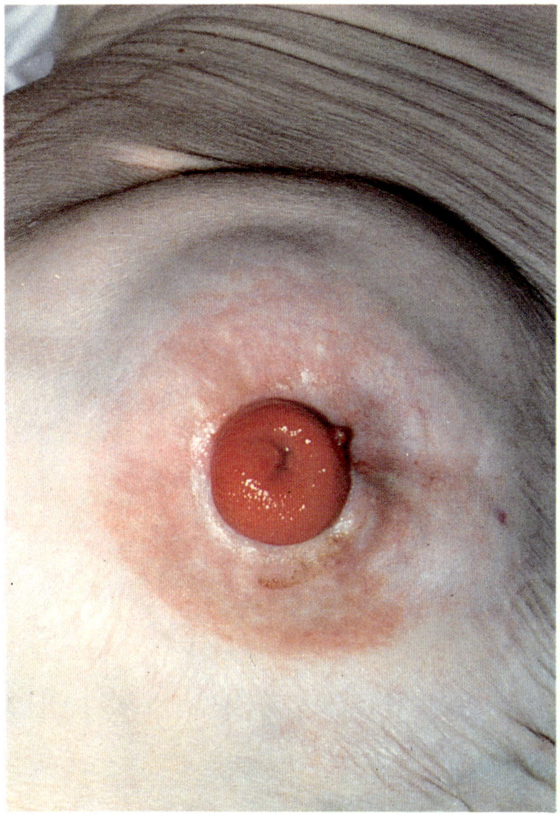

185 When lying, the hernia disappears but the stretched skin creates a fold that again hinders the fit of the appliance. Note the pyogenic granuloma resulting from trauma by the ill-fitting appliance.

186

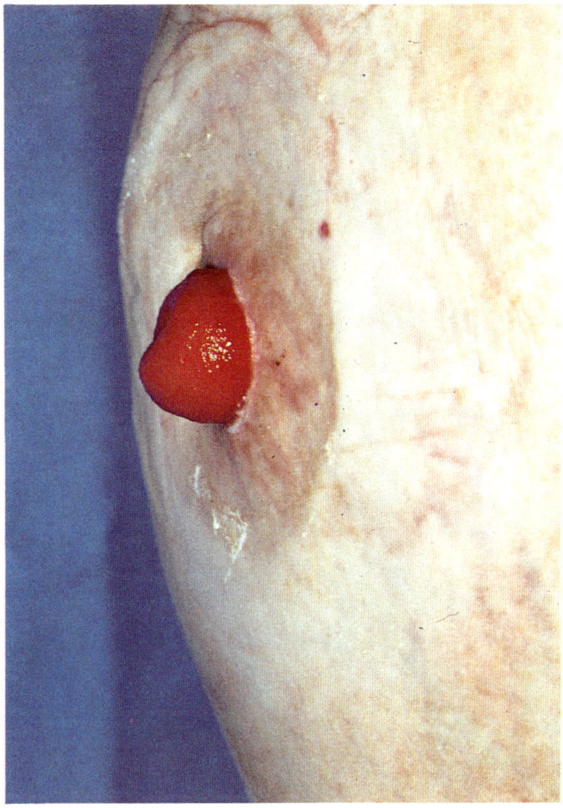

186 Three weeks after repair of the hernia via a superior circumstomal incision, with excision of redundant skin.

187

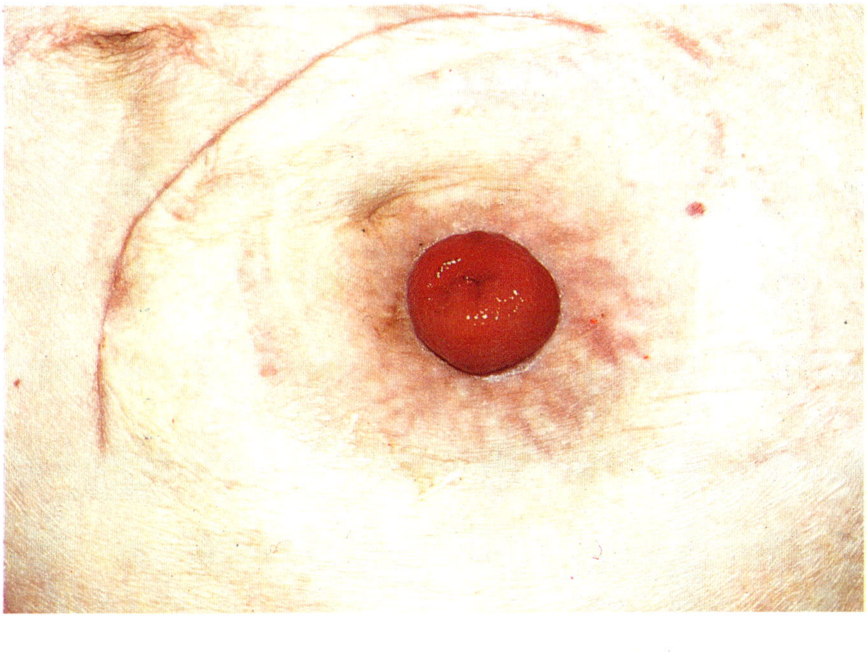

187 Already an improvement is evident in the peristomal skin.

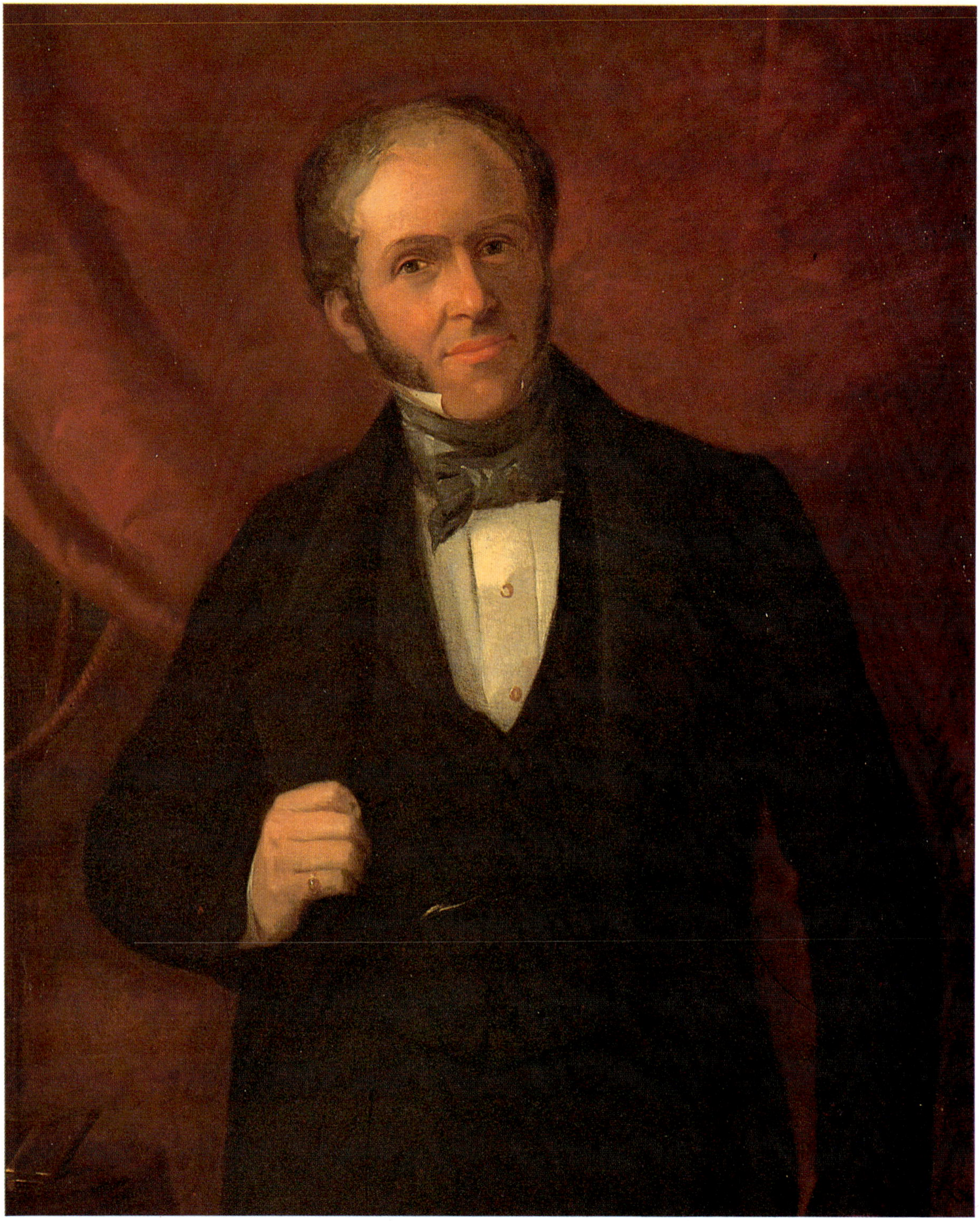

James Luke (1798–1881)
PRCS 1853 & 1862

First surgeon to fashion a sigmoid colostomy through a pararectal incision, in 1850
(Courtesy of Royal College of Surgeons of England)

Section III: Appliances and Accessories

Past appliances

The advances made in stoma appliances since the mid 1960s can only be appreciated in terms of what was available before the era of the odour-proof plastic sheet and the evolution of seals, wafers and adhesives to protect the skin. These advances have resulted from the efforts of industry, under the guidance of compassionate surgeons, striving to improve products with the patient's welfare foremost in mind.

Today's appliances are so different from those that were available at the dawn of stoma surgery, that it is worth remembering these early efforts and some of them are reproduced here to give historical continuity to the achievements in the development of the stoma armamentarium.

188

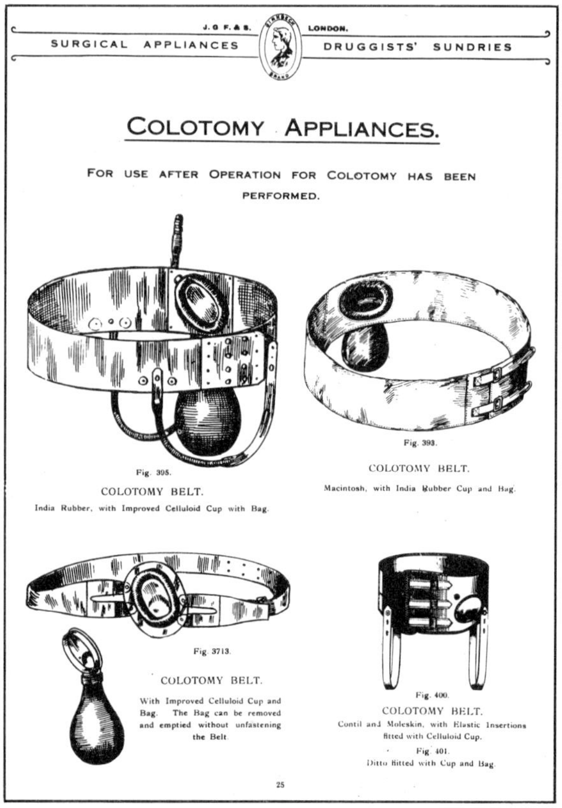

188 A page from a pre-1940 catalogue

The early appliances had to be strapped to the patient by belts. They followed the principles used in incontinence urinals.

They had to be tight to prevent seepage. Fabric, though comfortable, was easily soiled, and rubber was preferred because it was easier to wash. It had many drawbacks not least of all its smell, the sweat rash it produced, and the fact that the belt would ride up when sitting. Understraps had thus to be incorporated at times. To minimise the effects of sweating, rubber belts were perforated and lined with fleece.

Most belts needed to be unfastened to empty the appliance, though some carried detachable cups and bags. They were cumbersome, heavy and noticeable. Patients were self-conscious about them. Plugs were therefore devised in an effort to do away with some of their bulkiness.

The illustration is a typical selection of the various appliances in use for colostomies. None were very suitable for ileostomies.

The all india-rubber colostomy belt, with cup and bag of the same material (top, right) was suitable for bath use; while the wider belt in Contil (bottom, right) with a waterproof front section was for everyday or formal use.

189

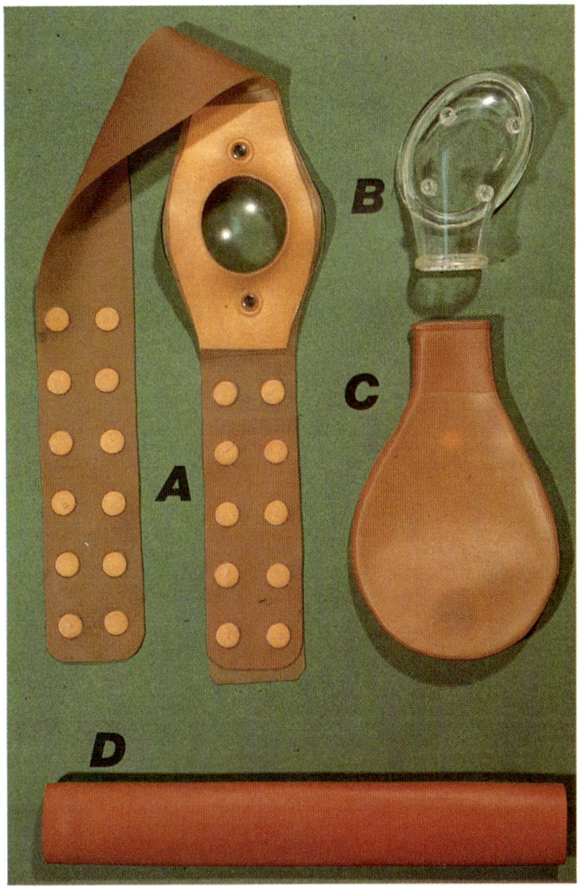

189 Colostomy appliance circa 1950.

A The typical rubber belt with a frontal aperture into which a celluloid cup fits. The latter carries two studs that can be pressed into corresponding holes on either side of the aperture. The cup is thus steadied by the studs, but can be easily slipped out for emptying or cleansing.

B A colostomy cup with chute made of celluloid. It had a solid rim with four studs at the back, was oval and so inclined as to be worn on the right, the left or centrally. The cups usually came in two sizes, medium or large.

C Rubber bag to fit to the chute of the above cup. The lower part of the bag on its posterior face carried an outlet for emptying.

D The chute could be fitted with a wide rubber tubing for wash-out or lavage.

190

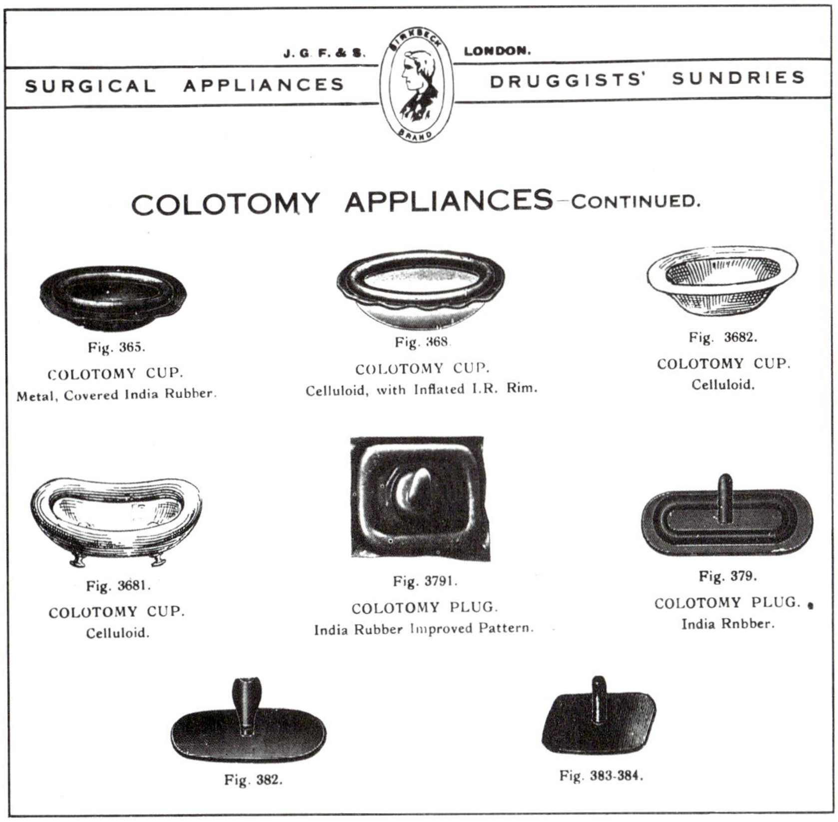

190 Various colostomy cups and plugs.

Cups came in various shapes to fit the abdominal curvature of thin, normal and obese patients. The rims were solid, hollow or in sponge rubber. They were round or oval. Originally, they were made of celluloid, but later on of plastic.

Plugs were made of soft or vulcanised rubber. They were mounted on a flat base, standing at right angles to it, or obliquely. For a closer fit some had a soft rim or flange. In many ways they were the precursors of the magnetic plug (Maclet).

191

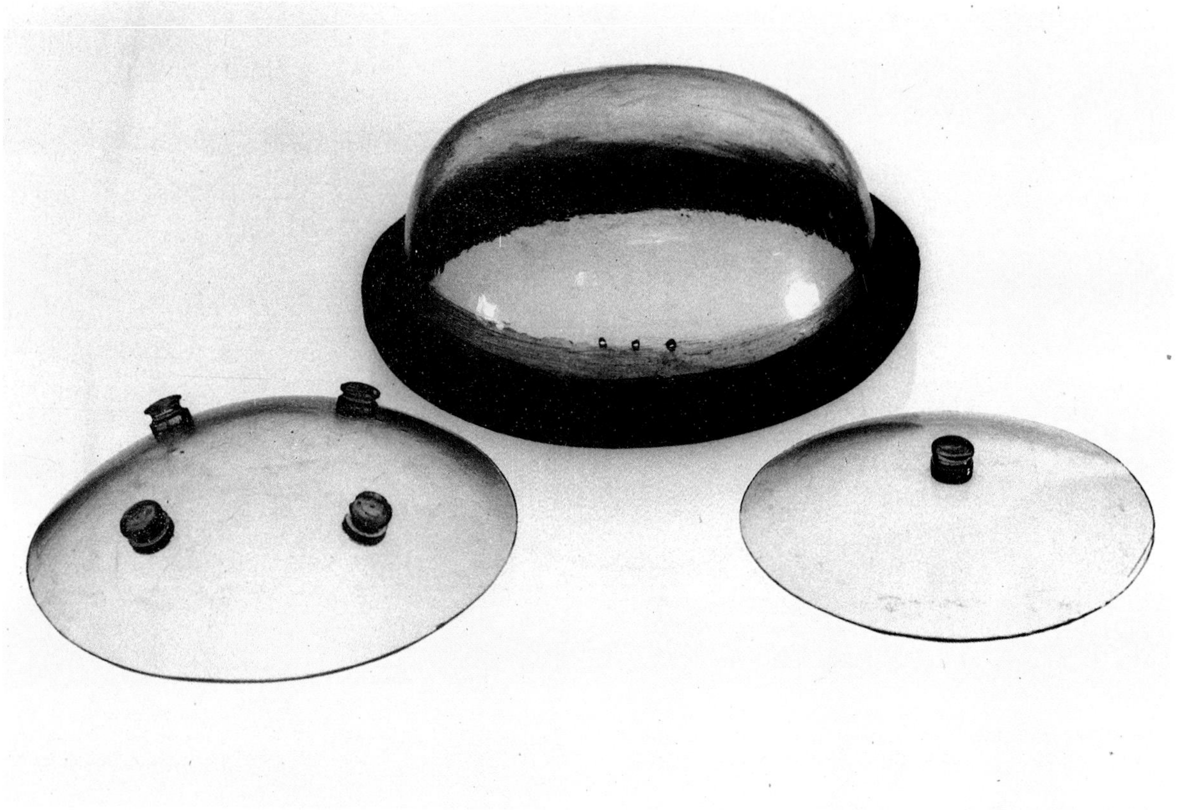

192

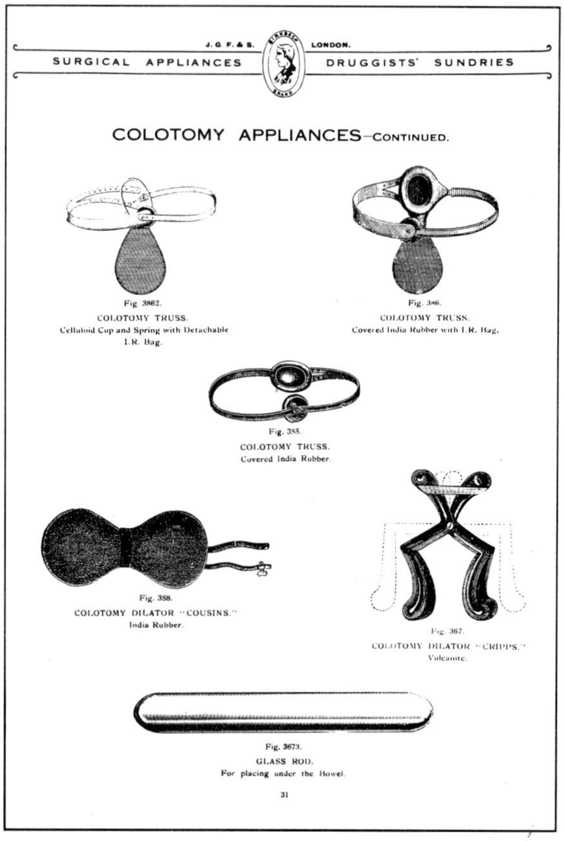

J. G. F. & S. LONDON.

SURGICAL APPLIANCES DRUGGISTS' SUNDRIES

COLOTOMY APPLIANCES—CONTINUED.

Fig. 3862.
COLOTOMY TRUSS.
Celluloid Cup and Spring with Detachable I.R. Bag.

Fig. 386.
COLOTOMY TRUSS.
Covered India Rubber with I.R. Bag.

Fig. 385.
COLOTOMY TRUSS.
Covered India Rubber.

Fig. 388.
COLOTOMY DILATOR "COUSINS."
India Rubber.

Fig. 367.
COLOTOMY DILATOR "CRIPPS."
Vulcanite.

Fig. 3673.
GLASS ROD.
For placing under the Bowel.

31

191 Cup and shields.

(1) A round colostomy cup with a hollow India-rubber rim. Note the three small perforations to let flatus out.
These cups were not odour-proof!

(2) Two St Mark's shields. They were supplied without studs, or with one, two or four studs. They were made of celluloid and came in various diameters up to five inches. They were ideal for casual wear, for use at night, or at such times as the colostomy was known not to work. Their flat domes were relatively inconspicuous under a garment and they were a better design than plugs.

192 Trusses and dilators.

The principles used in hernia trusses were applied to colostomy appliances and proved useful, except in obese patients. A bag or cup – or both – could be attached to them.

Strictures and stenoses were commonplace before the Brooke's stoma. They required daily dilatations. Dilators were of all types. Here an inflatable one and a cross-action one are depicted. Note the solid glass rod supplied for loop colostomies.

Modern types of appliances

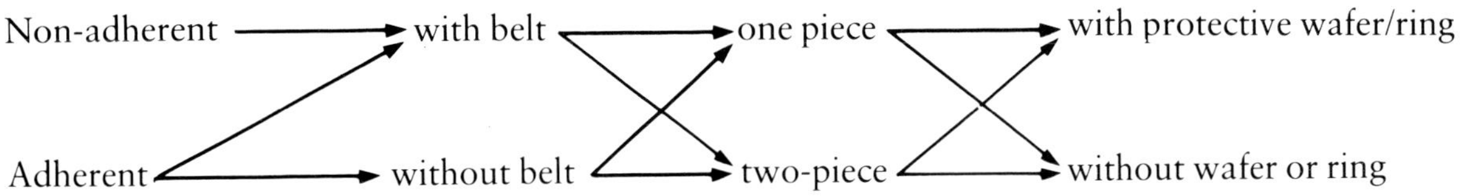

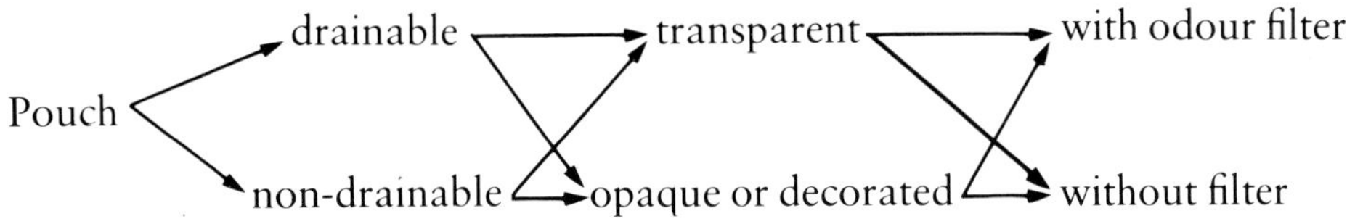

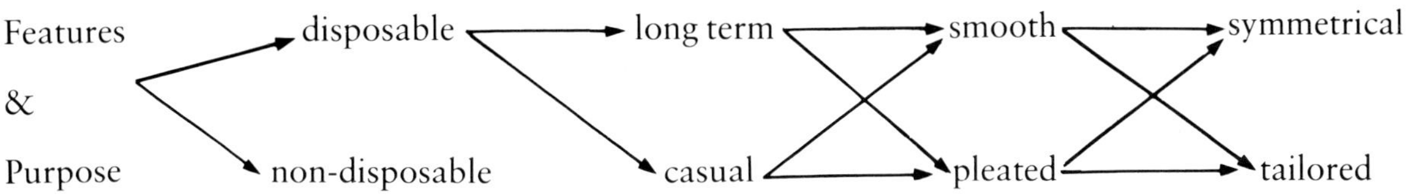

193

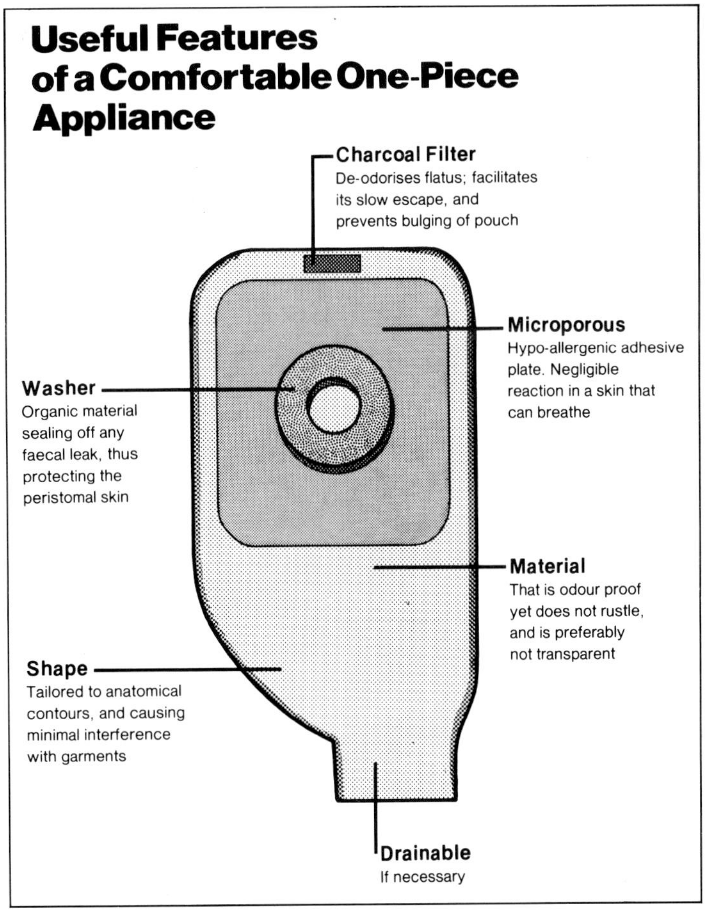

193 No appliance is ideal for every patient and situation – hence the great variety available. However, certain features contribute to a near-ideal situation, and industry has made enormous efforts at meeting the needs of all temperaments and body types. Here are outlined some useful features that will help the therapist in the choice of a good all-round one-piece appliance for long term use.

In the immediate post-operative period the features to look for are:

- A good adhesive faceplate, soft, and easy to apply and handle.
- Leakproof.
- Unlikely to generate skin problems.
- Odour-proof.
- Drainable, with a simple and safe clip.
- Transparent enough to allow good visualisation of the stoma.
- Inexpensive.
- Unobtrusive.

Appliances can be of one-piece, two-piece or three-piece types.

194

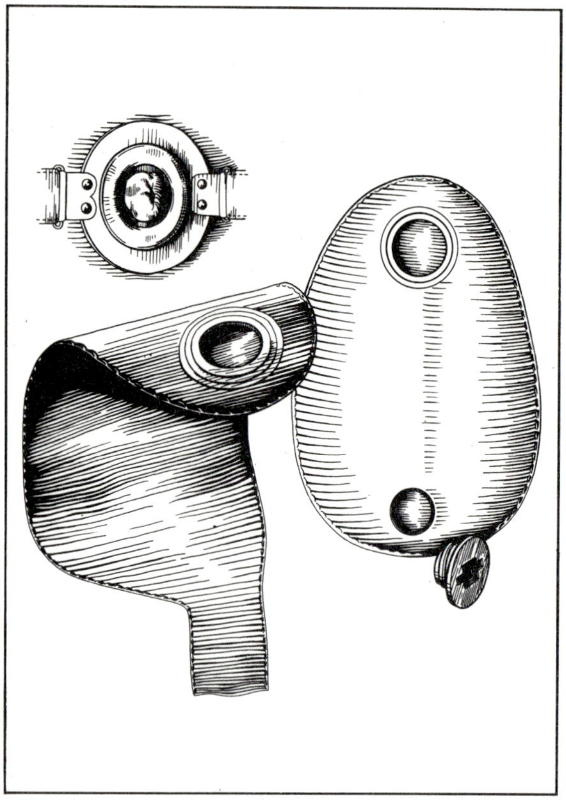

194 The Koenig Rutzen appliance was constructed in one piece, as was Salt's original modification which is still available (1986) and is made of odourproof black butyl or white rubber. A latex solution ensured leakproof adhesion of the facepiece of the skin. Down Bros. developed two-piece appliances, consisting of a flange made doubly secure by a belt.

A hole in the upper part of the bag fits tightly over the flange. The bag can thus be changed without disturbing the flange.

Bags have either a screw or a spout outlet, are washable and can be small or large. They are flat and do not rustle. Those used to them find them very secure. They could thus be described as non-adherent, in two pieces, with a belt and without a protective wafer (see p. 119). The bags are drainable and re-usable.

195

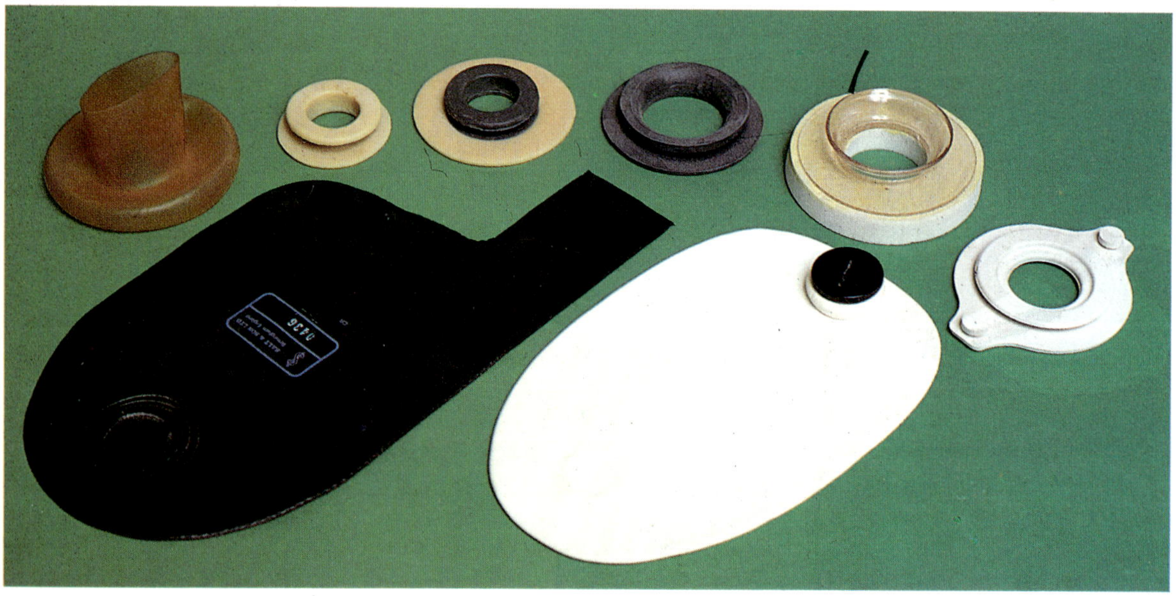

195 Two-piece type bags in black butyl or white rubber with a variety of available flanges. The flanges from left to right are:

(a) Latex protective sheath.
(b) Soft rubber.
(c) Semi-rigid rubber.
(d) Hard black rubber.
(e) Rigid facepiece mounted on a latex foam diaphragm.
(f) Flexible recessed flange with studs for a belt.

196

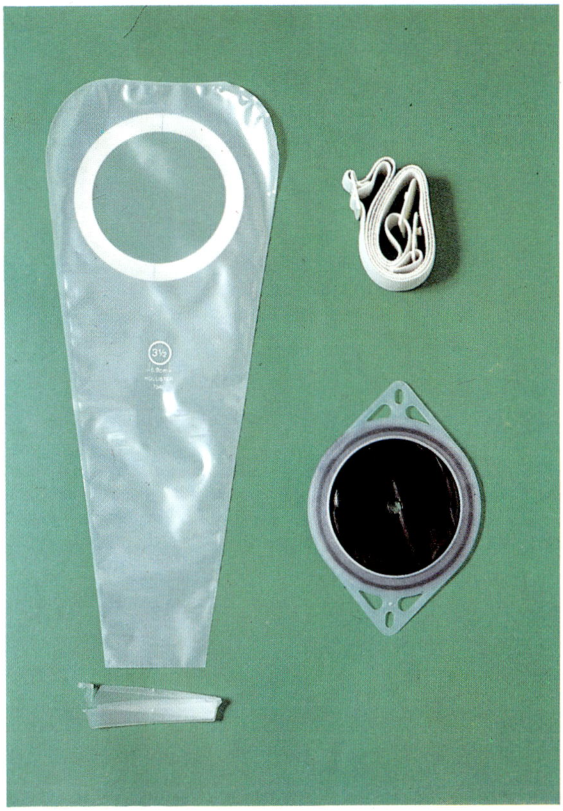

196 Example of a with-belt adherent appliance, in two pieces, carrying a combined protective wafer and ring. The pouch is transparent, drainable, and without a filter. It is smooth, symmetrical, disposable and of good length. These features, combined with a large ring and a wafer that can be ringed out to the size of the stoma, make it well suited for a defunctioning double-barrelled transverse colostomy.

197

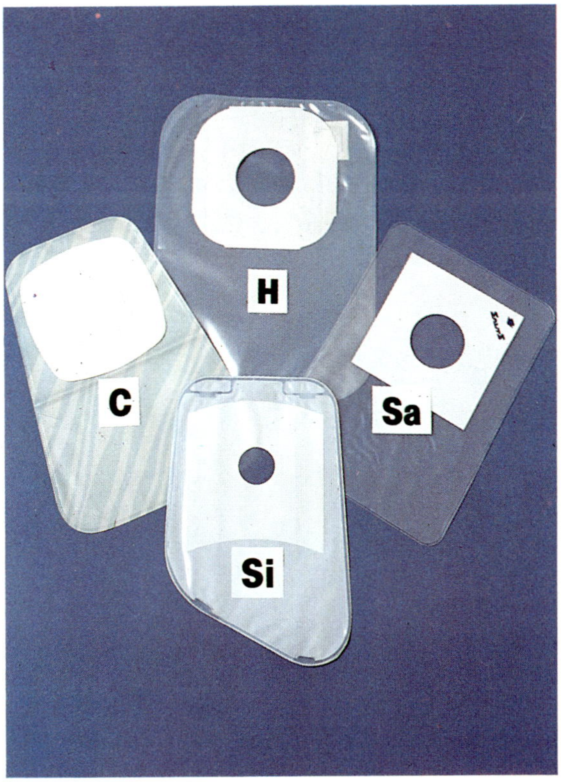

197 Adherent, without belt, one-piece appliances without wafer or ring. These are ideal for the fully stabilised patient with a colostomy. Once the colostomy has acted, appliance and contents can be disposed of.

198

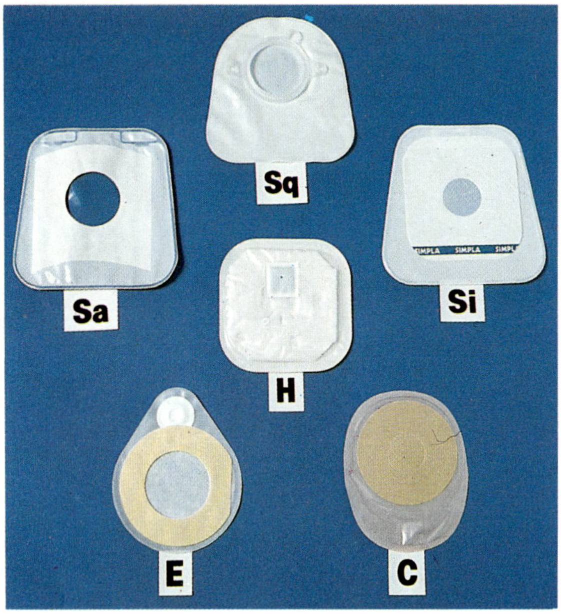

198 Similar appliances for 'casual' wear. They are smaller, will not show through a thin dress or swim suit; they can be worn when the colostomy is known not to be active, or for dancing, sporting activities, or during intercourse.

Sq is worn with a belt over a ring and wafer.

H and E carry filter pads.

Protective rings

These have become a feature of 'second generation' appliances. Two main types are encountered based on their major constituents, which are:

(a) Karaya gum.

(b) Methyl cellulose derivatives with or without polyisobutylene (PIB).

A. *Karaya*

This is a natural polysaccharide gum derived from plants of the Sterculia family found in India. It will dry up as a powder which is beige to grey-pink, but will change to a brown or dark brown colour when treated. It is slightly soluble in water, and is insoluble in alcohol or ether. It is highly hygroscopic and was initially used as a dental fixative powder.

As it absorbs water it becomes more and more gelatinous and soft, finally disintegrating. Glycerin is added to it when 'cured' into washers. The latter are produced either by dipping rings of lint in the gum, or simply cutting them out from sheets of the set gum.

Warmth and humidity soften the ring and allow it to be moulded around a stoma or inside hollows. Cold and dryness stiffen it, making it rigid. Thus a dry and cool place is ideal for storing the appliances, but before use the wafer should be warmed on a radiator or between the palms of the hands, or even wiped with a wet swab. It should be applied to dry skin that has been cleaned with soap and water but not with alcohol or ether.

B. *Methylcellulose derivatives*

Stomahesive is the best known product made from methycellulose derivatives but most manufacturers of appliances now have their own version of these compounds.

It is a mixture of gelatin, pectin, PIB and sodium carboxy methyl cellulose. Like Karaya gum it was first used in the mouth as a dental adhesive. It was initially produced in squares of 10 × 10 cm. It adheres naturally to skin whether dry or moist, and will mould itself to its contours. It can stay in position up to two weeks. It is comfortable, can be left *in situ* during a bath and affords remarkable protection to the skin. It is stiffer than karaya, and there are more malleable variants of it which have various advantages. As a group, these protective rings based on methylcellulose are remarkably anallergic.

Amongst these variants are Hollihesive, Comfeel held in an elastomeric framework, and Seel-a-peel which contains a particularly hydrophylic polymer, and is based on karaya gum.

199

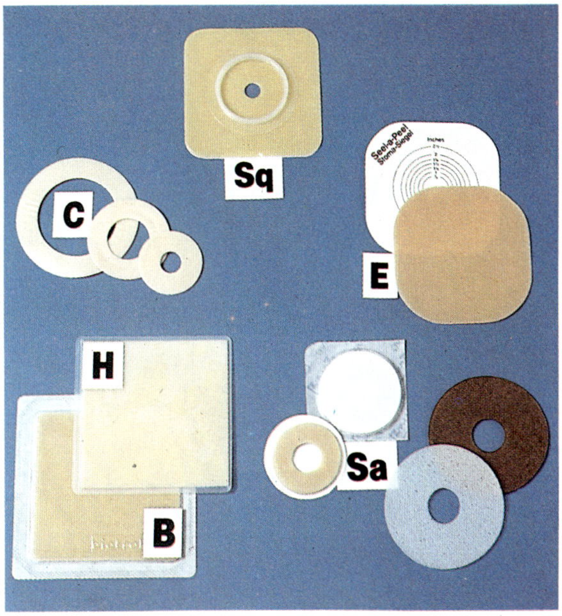

199 Shows a variety of such protective rings or squares, the lettering indicating their source (see p. 137).

Drainable systems with seals

Adjustable apertures allow the patient to keep to a single system during the early days of training – days during which frequent aperture adjustments are often necessary. However, it puts the onus for using the correct aperture on the patient, and therefore some degree of pre-selection is advisable.

Eschmann Ltd have replaced the rings with a spiral which can be unwound to the required aperture, the unwanted portion being torn off or cut away. This is a convenient system, but requires a little patience.

Drainable systems demand reliable clips. Those shown here (**200, 201**) are very safe. The Hollister clip is curved to follow abdominal contours, and is therefore less obtrusive. This could also be achieved by using a shorter clip, but this would then narrow the outlet of the bag. The Eschmann clip is ingenious and easy to undo. It is, however, a little more conspicuous on thin patients.

Drainable systems are for use in patients with fluid stools, i.e. in the immediate post-operative period, in ileostomies, and in the event of diarrhoea.

Fixed aperture seals need a slightly thicker karaya ring than the adjustable variety; Coloplast produces one of the thinnest cushions. The Hollister seal seems the most hygroscopic and does not need moistening before application.

Round adhesive faceplates seem to catch less on clothing and to peel off less frequently than square ones.

200

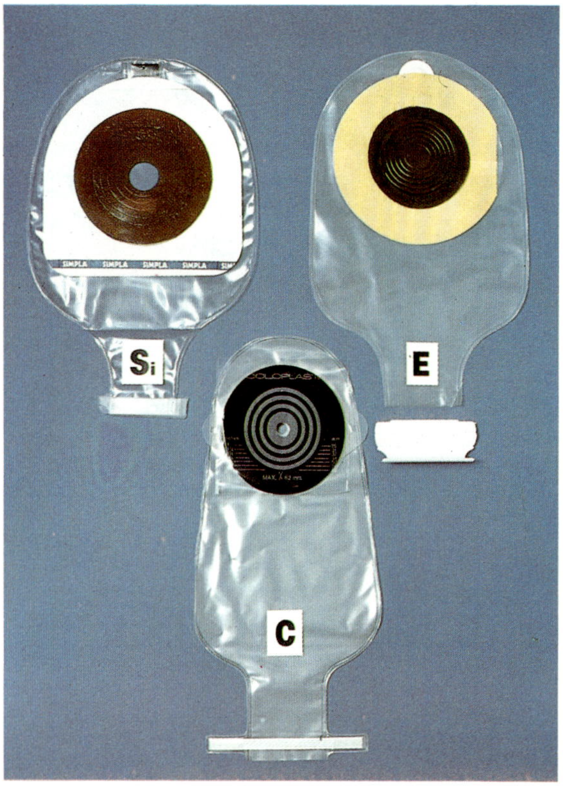

200 Karaya seals with adjustable apertures. A series of rings marked out on the karaya gum seal allows the correct aperture to be chosen. A finger is inserted under the seal to the appropriate size ring and the unwanted rings peeled out.

201

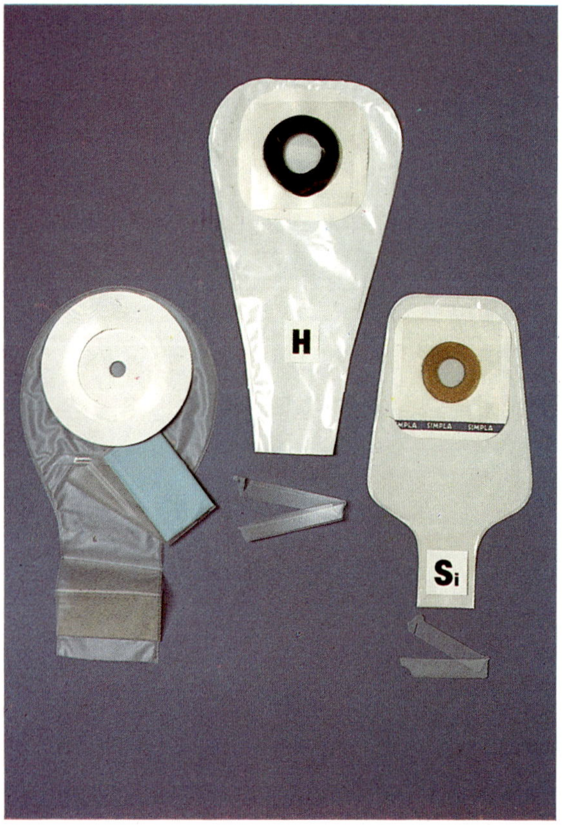

201 Seals with fixed apertures. Seals with varying size apertures are the commonest; the patient is guided through the necessary changes until the permanent size has been reached.

Note the system of outlet closure in the Salt pouch (unlabelled). The outlet proper is folded over itself several times and tucked into a rectangular pocket that fits it tightly. It is secure yet inconspicuous, will not show through covering garments, and cannot be felt.

202

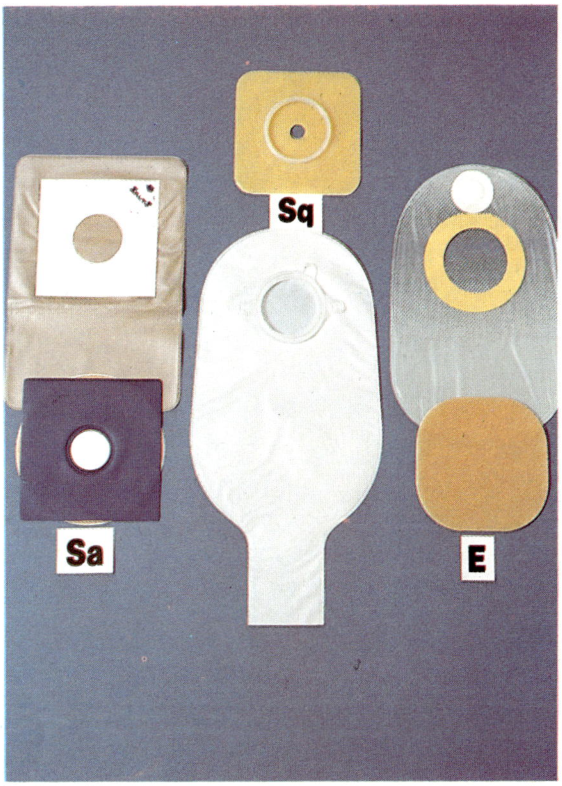

202 Two-piece appliances used with a plate or ring. **Sa** and **E** are of the adherent variety, the pouch carrying an adhesive backing that fixes on to a plate stuck to the abdominal skin. **Sq** uses a ring and belt system to achieve the same end.

These appliances are useful in the early days of a colostomy when stools are still fluid, or in an ileostomy. They allow frequent changes of the pouch without damage to the skin. All distraction takes place between pouch and plate only. Patients like the 2-piece appliances as they are less traumatic to change.

Appliances for double barrel or large colostomies

203

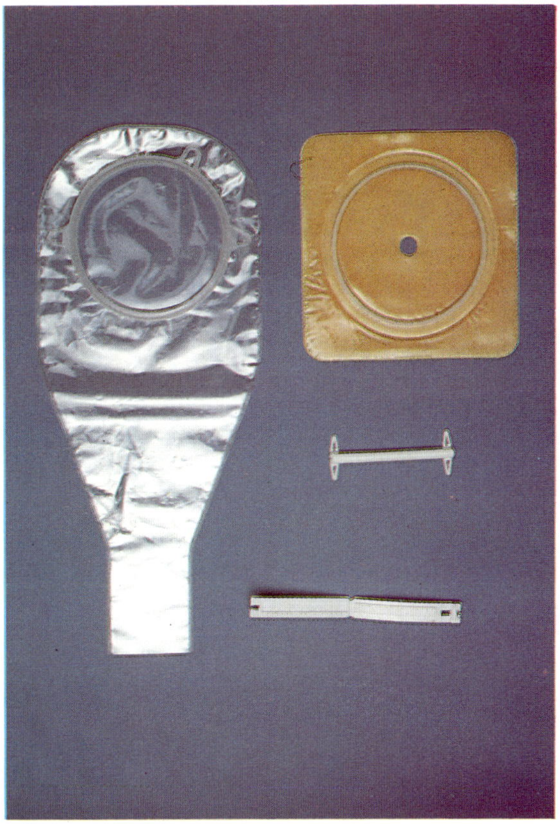

203 A large ring carried on an adherent wafer allows the plate aperture to be tailored to the size of the stoma, however large. It can accommodate the colostomy support with ease.

The pouch is of ample size with a funnelled lower end to facilitate drainage of a fluid stool. The pouch can be emptied at regular intervals to decrease its weight and minimise traction on the wafer and skin; or can be discarded and replaced.

204

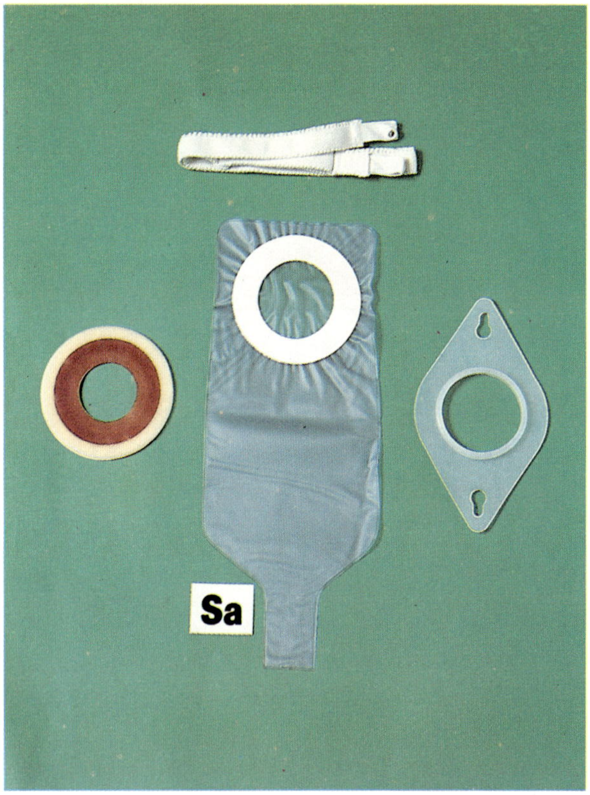

204 A three-piece appliance for a similar purpose. An adherent wafer held down by a plate secured by a belt provides a good seal for a pouch with an adhesive backing. The pouch can thus be emptied when full, or disposed of without disturbing plate seal or skin. Such appliances can be syringed with water to wash down their contents, but the manoeuvre is cumbersome and not specially cherished by patients who find it pleasanter to treat the pouch as a 'one use' disposable.

205

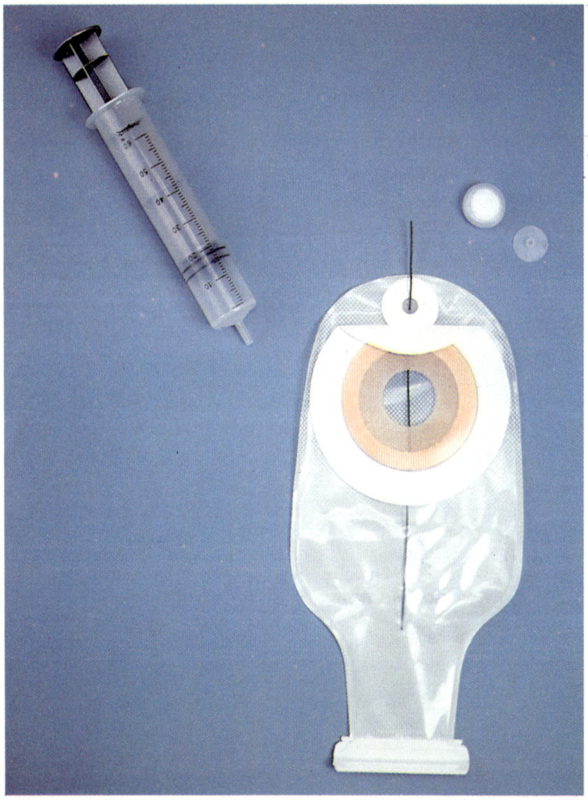

205 Eschmann have overcome this difficulty by an ingenious device. They have reinforced the filter hole at the top of the appliance so that it can carry either a small plastic bung or a filter pad. At the same time they have made the hole wide enough to accept the nozzle of a syringe. The patient can thus wash through the appliance from above without disturbing it and can change from bung to filter as convenient, giving a variety of options.

Filters, though useful in avoiding the embarrassment of a pouch suddenly filling up with flatus can, if too powerful, cause negative pressure within the pouch, leading the walls to stick so that stools will not drop. The filter may then become contaminated or wet and fail to function.

206

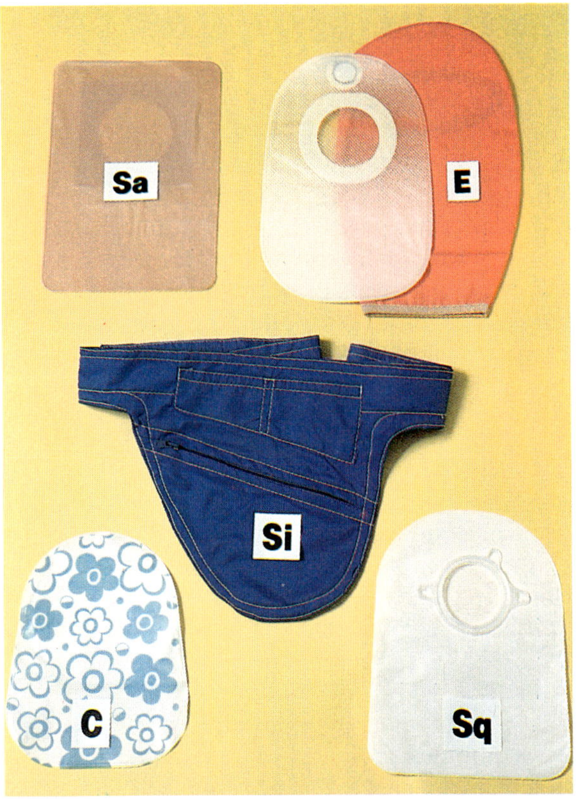

206 Opaque and coloured pouches. Pouch covers.

Some patients feel ill at ease with transparent pouches, especially in more intimate domestic surroundings. Opaque white and tinted pouches, as well as colourful ones are available for such circumstances. Alternatively, simple covers (E) or covers with a belt and pocket can discretely hide the contents of a transparent bag and appliance. Beige pouches tend to show less under clothing than a white or coloured ones.

SKIN PROTECTIVES, CLEANSING AGENTS AND DEODORANTS

Once excoriated, skin becomes very sore and will suffer further damage if an adhesive backed plate is applied to it. It needs to be covered either by a protective film, or by a paste barrier. Some preparations are also soothing, usually by their cooling effect. Protective film is available in aerosol form, as surgical wipes, as 'gel' or as lotions which can be painted on. Soap remains the best agent for cleaning the skin around a stoma; scented soap adds to the sensation of cleanliness. Deodorants in conveniently small containers are marketed by several stoma appliance companies.

207

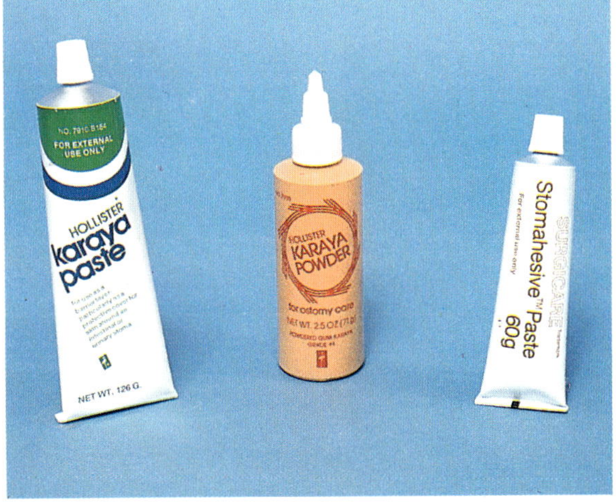

207 Pastes are supplied in small tubes of convenient size to be carried in a hand bag or jacket pocket. They are easily applied with the little finger to fill in recesses or to be smoothed over a sore area. Powders are more suitable for use at home and are usually hygroscopic.

Appendix

Adhesives and adhesive removers

Many adhesives are of medical silicone formula with little if any allergenic properties. They come as aerosol sprays or as easily spread solutions. They offer extra adhesion to a plate, minimise 'drag', and prevent leakage.

If a plate is used it should not be peeled away without the help of an adhesive remover as otherwise the outer epidermal cells will be repeatedly stripped and excoriation will result.

Irrigation therapy

Intermittent irrigation has regained popularity in recent years. Depending on the activity of the colon and the patient's occupation, irrigation is carried out daily or on alternate days. After emptying most of the colon, an appliance is not necessary and the patient wears at the most a casual pouch, and usually only a stoma cap.

Irrigation is ideal for young active adults mentally and physically capable of coping with the problems of irrigation. It requires time, competence, a well formed spout, good home toilet facilities and nimble fingers. It is imperative that the patient be clearly instructed in its use, and not allowed to go home until fully conversant and fully competent in handling the equipment. A catheter is not advisable for irrigation as perforation has been reported. Instead, a fairly soft plastic cone jammed into the stoma is preferable.

208

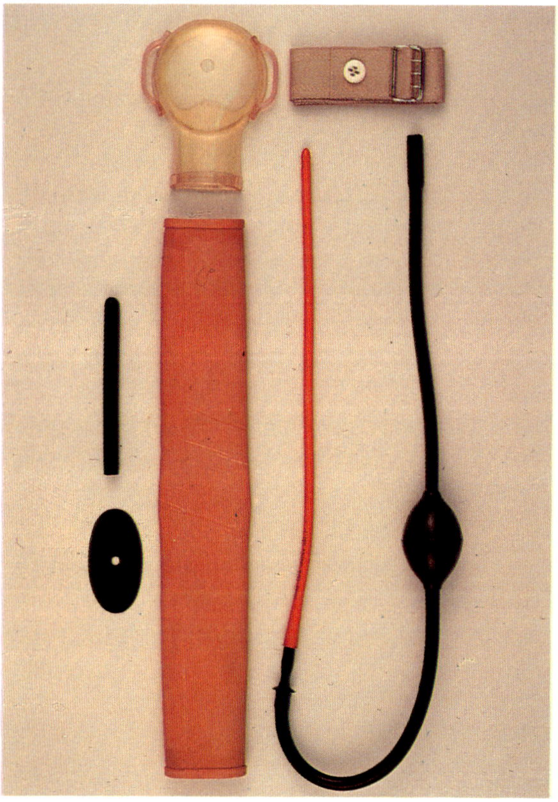

208 Colostomy lavage is not new; it was frequently used in the early days of stoma surgery.

This figure shows the Mitchell pattern dating back to the mid 1950s. It consisted of a celluloid chute held in place by a belt. The dome of the chute was holed to allow the passage of a rubber catheter through which lavage was carried out using a Higginson enema pump. If this was used without a catheter, an oval black india rubber washer acted as a guard. A wide rubber flat tubing fixed to the lower opening of the chute drained all returning fluid into a bucket. Any residual fluid was finally drained using a short black india rubber tube.

209

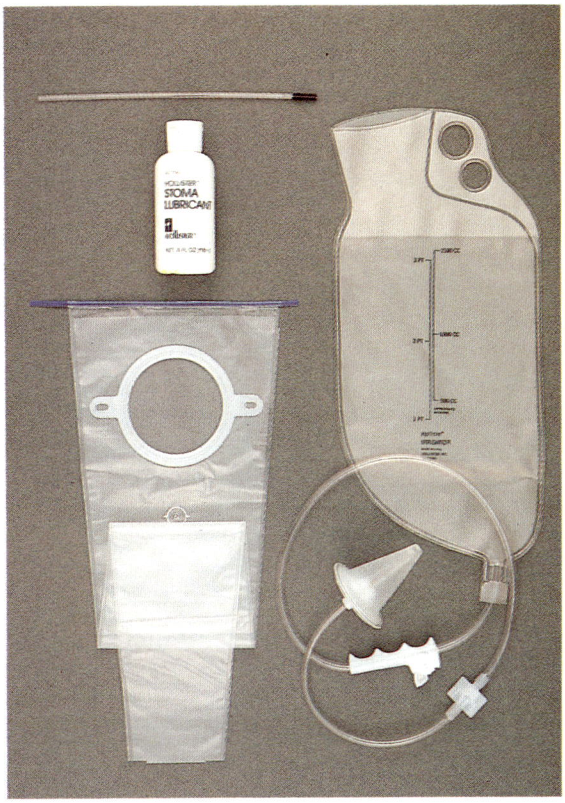

209 The modern version of an irrigation set. The plastic collecting bag is open at both ends, the upper one being wide enough to accept all manipulations. Irrigation is from a large plastic bag held at adjustable levels and carrying a long delivery tube controlled by a roller clip. A conical device held firmly into the stomal lumen delivers the irrigation fluid. A cleaning brush and a bottle of lubricating gel complete the set.

Effects of drugs on stomas

It can be argued that most drugs affect the gastro-intestinal tract; what will be discussed here are those drugs most likely to alter stoma function, and the effects which need to be drawn to the attention of the clinician and stoma therapist so that the patient may be enlighted and reassured. Unlike a normal patient with a sphincter and with a colon to re-absorb water, a patient with a stoma has no control over intestinal action and, therefore, is aware of side effects that normally would not be apparent.

Drugs affect the gastrointestinal tract in three main ways:

(a) Direct action on the gut.

(b) Action via neurotransmitters.

(c) Indirect action either via the central nervous system or by their effect on other organs, eg kidneys.

(a) *Direct action on the gut*

Most purgatives and most constipating agents belong to this group, and are used when their therapeutic effect is desired. Morphine, codeine, dihydrocodeine and diphenoxylate are useful constipating agents. However, constipation is an undesirable side effect of morphine and dihydrocodeine when they are used as analgesics. Dextropropoxyphene and buprenorphine are less constipating analgesics. Loperamide belongs to the next group of drugs as it works probably via its action on cholinergic and non-cholinergic transmitters.

Antacids based on magnesium will increase looseness, whereas those containing calcium and aluminium have the reverse effect.

Antibiotics will alter gut flora and may cause monilial invasion of the gut, with distressing diarrhoea, as well as peristomal soreness.

(b) *Action via neuro-transmitters*

The gut has adrenergic, dopaminergic and cholinergic receptors.

Cholinergic stimulation increases peristaltic and secretory activity, but decreases sphincter tone. Drugs blocking cholinergic activity will have the reverse effect in that they dry up secretion and cause constipation.

Sympathetic stimulation via adrenergic and dopaminergic transmission tends to oppose cholinergic activity. Thus noradrenaline and dopamine will decrease peristalsis, but whereas the former causes vasoconstriction, the latter is a vasodilator.

Anticholinergic drugs in frequent use are atropine, hyoscine and the belladonna group; propantheline and poldine in anti-peptic ulcer treatment; dicyclomine as an anti-emetic or anti-spasmodic; and emepromium for urinary instability in the elderly.

Cholinergic drugs such as bethanecol and neostigmine may cause intestinal colic and diarrhoea.

Many commonly used drugs have anti-cholinergic properties. In this group are most of the compounds used in the treatment of parkinsonism; the phenothiazines, notably chlorpromazine (its anticholinergic activity being stronger than its α-adrenergic blocking properties), many tricyclic antidepressants and most antihistamines. Some cardiac drugs used for the correction of dysrhythmia, e.g. quinine and disopyramide, have also anti-cholinergic effects. Drugs competing with acetylcholine such as the ganglion-blocking agents will cause constipation.

Anti-adrenergic drugs are more commonly used than adrenergic ones.

Alpha-adrenergic blockade by drugs such as thymoxamine has been tried in the treatment of peripheral vascular disease. It causes diarrhoea. Similarly, drugs blocking nor-adrenaline release, such as guanethidine, will have the same effect. Reserpine depletes tissues of stored adrenaline; methyldopa prevents conversions of dopa to dopamine – the precursor of noradrenaline – and thus exhibits anti-adrenergic effects on the gut.

(c) *Indirect action via other organs or tissues*

Diuretics are not infrequently used in the post-operative period. Their effect on the volume of extracellular fluids and on the sodium/potassium requirements of smooth muscle can lead to constipation.

So also can sedatives and anxiolytic drugs. Their constipating action is probably a central one influencing parasympathetic tone, and distinct from any direct anticholinergic effects that some may have.

Digoxin will cause diarrhoea, and this too is thought to be a central action – but the mechanism is unclear. The patient who cannot do without digoxin will then require a constipatory agent.

Unless a drug needs to be given to a patient (with a stoma) for a clear therapeutic purpose, for a predetermined period and to a conclusive result, the clinician would be well advised to avoid any empirical therapy and any useless placebo effect in this group of patients.

DIET, MEALS AND STOMAS

There is no such thing as an ileostomy or colostomy diet. Each individual behaves differently and sometimes has to learn his or her own bodily foibles. However, some types of foods affect the effluent in a specific way and it is advisable to give the patient a general idea of what to expect, and when.

An ileostomy is at its most active about an hour after a meal; and the larger the meal the greater the activity. Since many people have their main meal at the end of the day during the working week, their ileostomy may be most active in the evening. On the other hand, a colostomy will usually tend to work after the first meal of the day or the morning cup of tea. In someone with a previous history of colonic spasticity, the colostomy may produce a soft or even a loose stool after every meal.

The gut cannot break down cellulose which is both bulky and holds on to water, producing a soft stool. Foodstuffs with a high cellulose content should therefore be avoided or be eaten sparingly in the beginning.

Fizzy drinks and gas-forming foods; i.e. pulses, will give a sensation of bloatedness and will increase gas evacuation, so patients should be cautioned against overindulgence in them. Gas may be with or without odour, and can increase peristaltic activity and mimick a laxative. Some foods can be constipating and gas-inhibiting as well as odour-reducing.

210

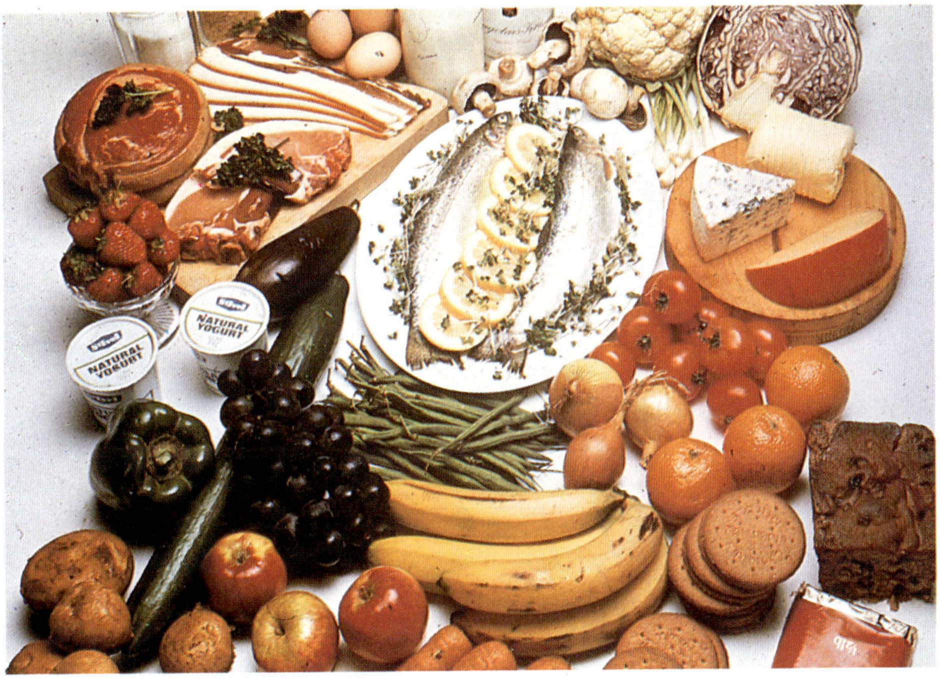

210 shows a variety of foods in everyday consumption that can be used to test a patient's knowledge of how they affect a colostomy.

Eggs, mushrooms and fish produce odour; cauliflower, cabbage, onions, green beans, cucumber and green pepper can produce wind. Yoghurt inhibits gas formation.

Hard cheese, fruit cake, chocolate and nuts, bananas, carrots, apples and aubergines are constipating.

Starchy foods such as biscuits, potatoes and rice are recommended in moderation, as are lean meat and soft fresh fruit. Blue cheeses, venison, smoked fish and mayonnaise are best avoided to start with, but can gradually be introduced in the diet.

Figs, prunes, beer, fresh milk and spinach can all have a mild laxative effect and should be indulged in sparingly.

211

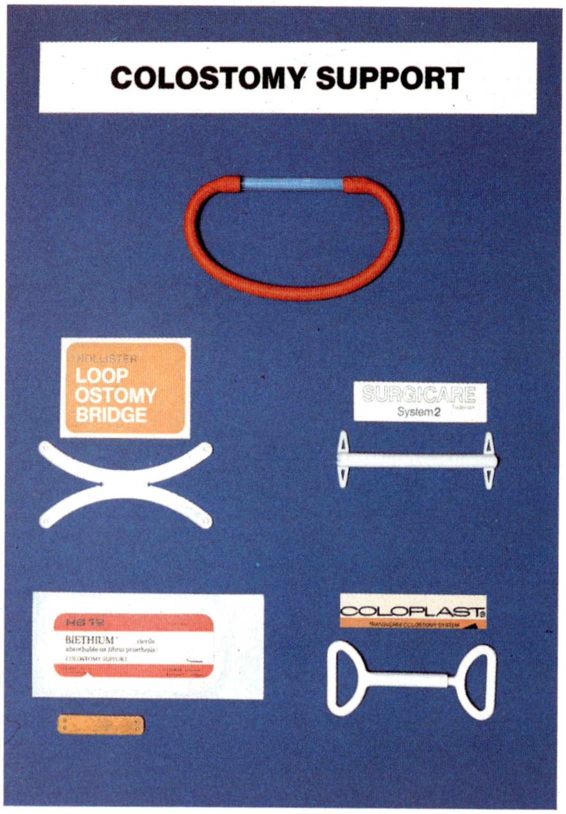

211 A range of colostomy supports supplied by various appliance manufacturers. The old-fashioned glass rod with rubber tubing still has its proponents; the degradable oxfibrin rod – Biethium – is an elegant way of supporting a temporary loop colostomy.

212

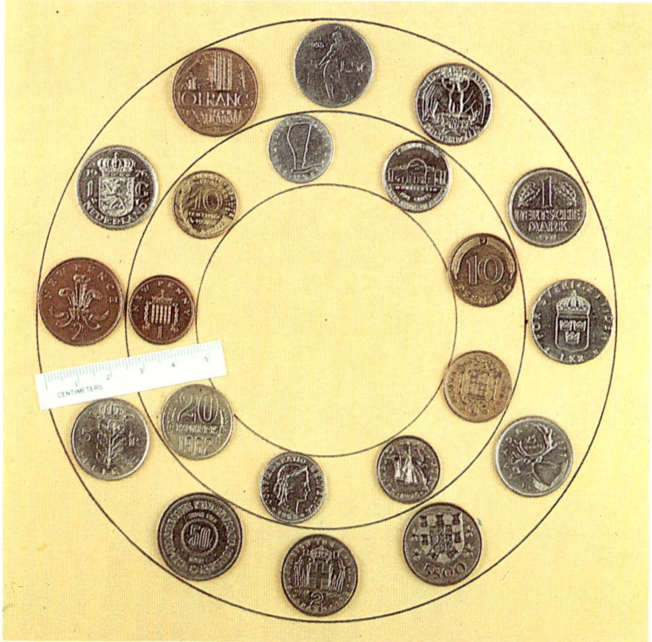

212 A collection of coins of various countries showing sizes very similar to the penny or 2p of the UK coinage, with the actual size in centimetres.

Two varieties of monofilament suture ideally suited for subcuticular stitching.

213

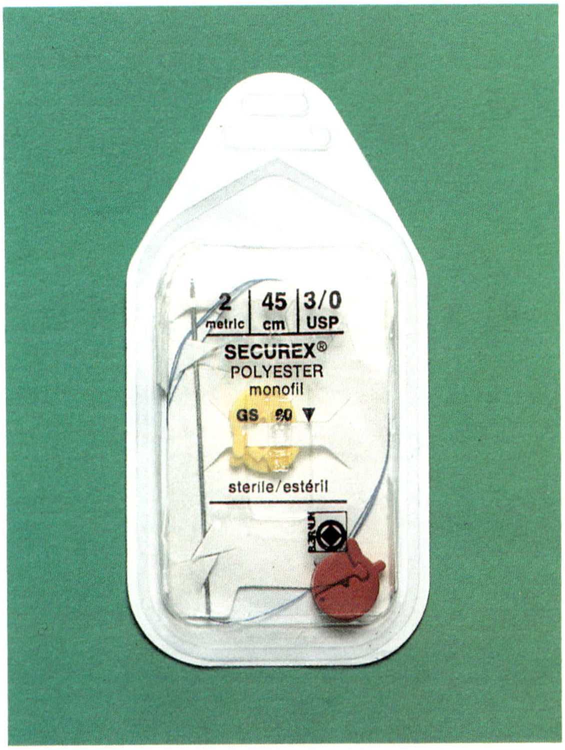

213 Polyester suture, made by Braun of Germany (supplied in the UK by Davis & Geck) has adjustable buttons, which avoids the discomfort caused by too taut a stitch made worse by swelling in the immediate post-operative period.

214

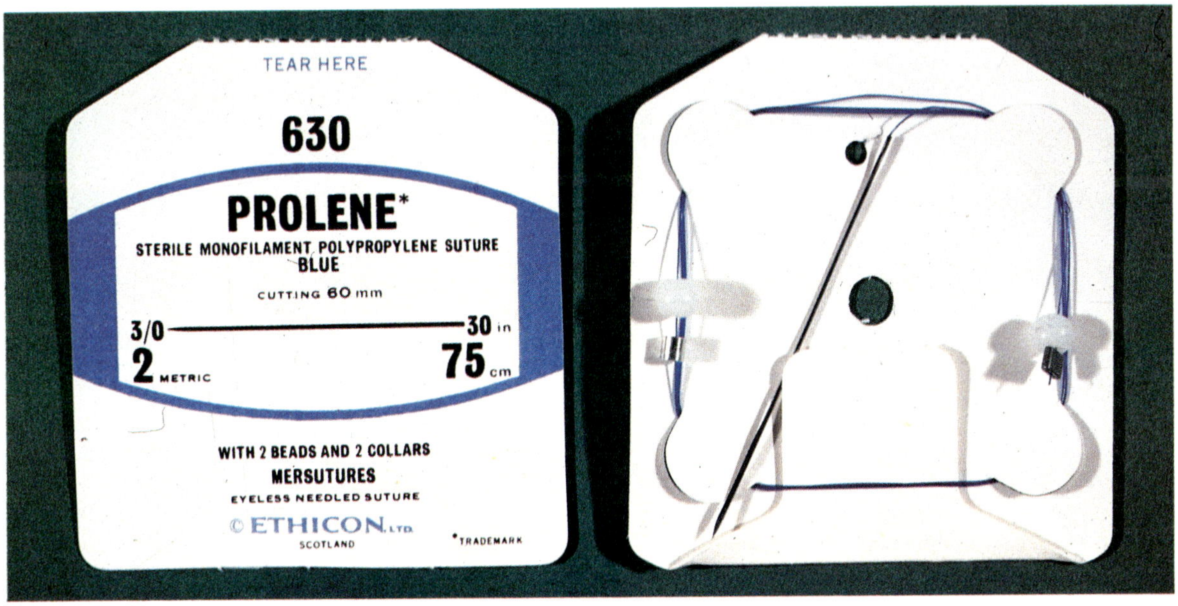

214 Polyurethane suture, made by Ethicon, has fixed beads and comes in a useful 75 cm length.

215

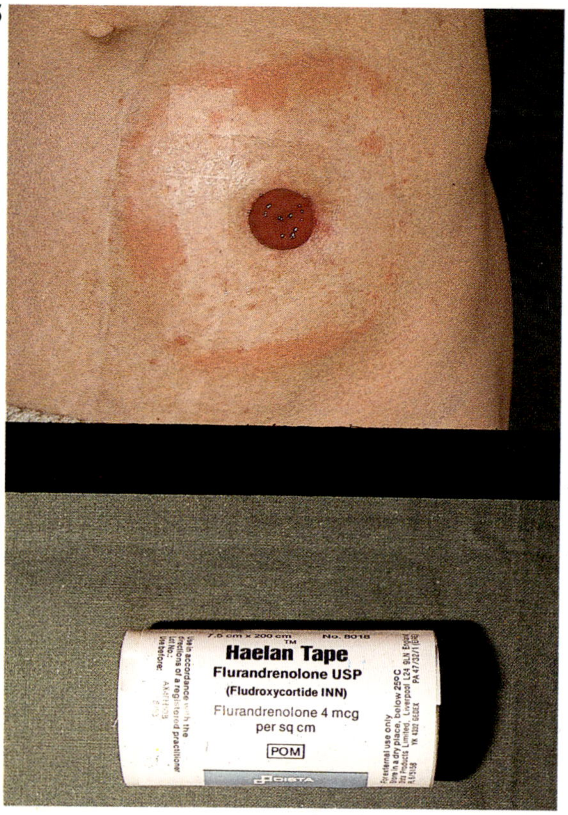

215 A steroid impregnated tape useful for treating allergic reactions. The appliance can be fitted directly on to the reverse side of the tape and will stick securely to it.

216

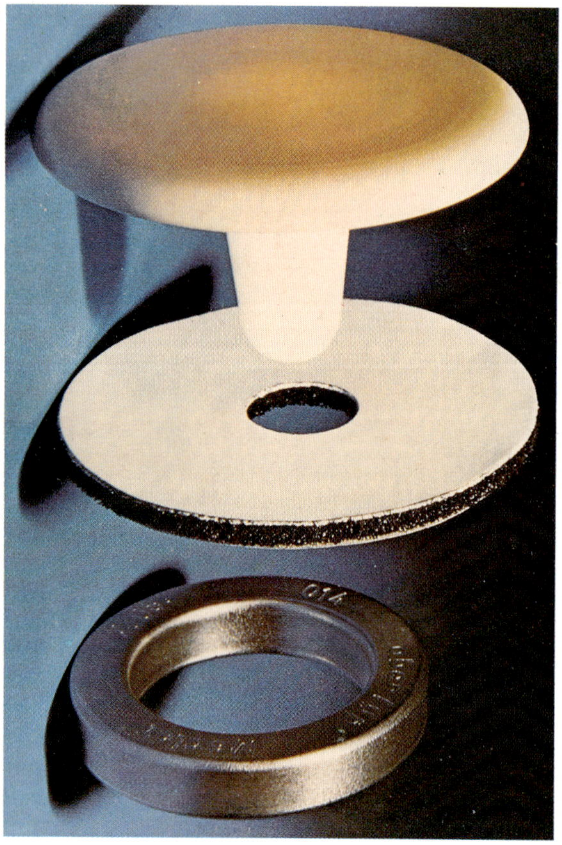

216 The Maclet magnetic device. The magnetic ring at the bottom is normally buried in the subcutaneous fat; the cap, above, is held within the stoma by its pin. It is drawn in by magnetic force. These caps are made of nylon or polyurethane and come with different lengths and diameters of pins to fit patients with varying thicknesses of fat or lengths of spout.

Industry has so far made great strides in resolving many of the problems that face the 'ostomate', such as the adhesive qualities of backing plates, contact allergy, odour proof material, rustling of pouches, and to a lesser extent, escape of flatus.

Spectacular advances are unlikely to be added to these efforts, although there is still room for improvement in the production of seamless bags with greater safety, as well as in the convenience of disposal and of changing of pouches, especially when the patient has to cope with non-domestic circumstances.

These aspects have led Trimark Medical to produce a new appliance still in its trial stages. The main feature of the device is a cylindrical bag with a usable length of two feet. The bag is seamless and packed tightly onto a spool or cassette from which any length can be dispensed as required. Once the dispensed portion has filled up it can be isolated, torn off and disposed of without disturbing the appliance. Another length of the film is then dispensed to start the process again. Thus, no smell need escape during the disposal manoeuvre.

Delivery of the film by this method amounts to the equivalent of five standard pouches, in addition to which the patient can dispense a length according to need; that is, less during inactive hours and more during overactive periods. Also, the two foot length allows the appliance to be used either for irrigation purposes or for low emptying direct into a pan. Additional features are a very secure double-lock clip; a high volume filter for flatus control, and the security of a seamless film.

217

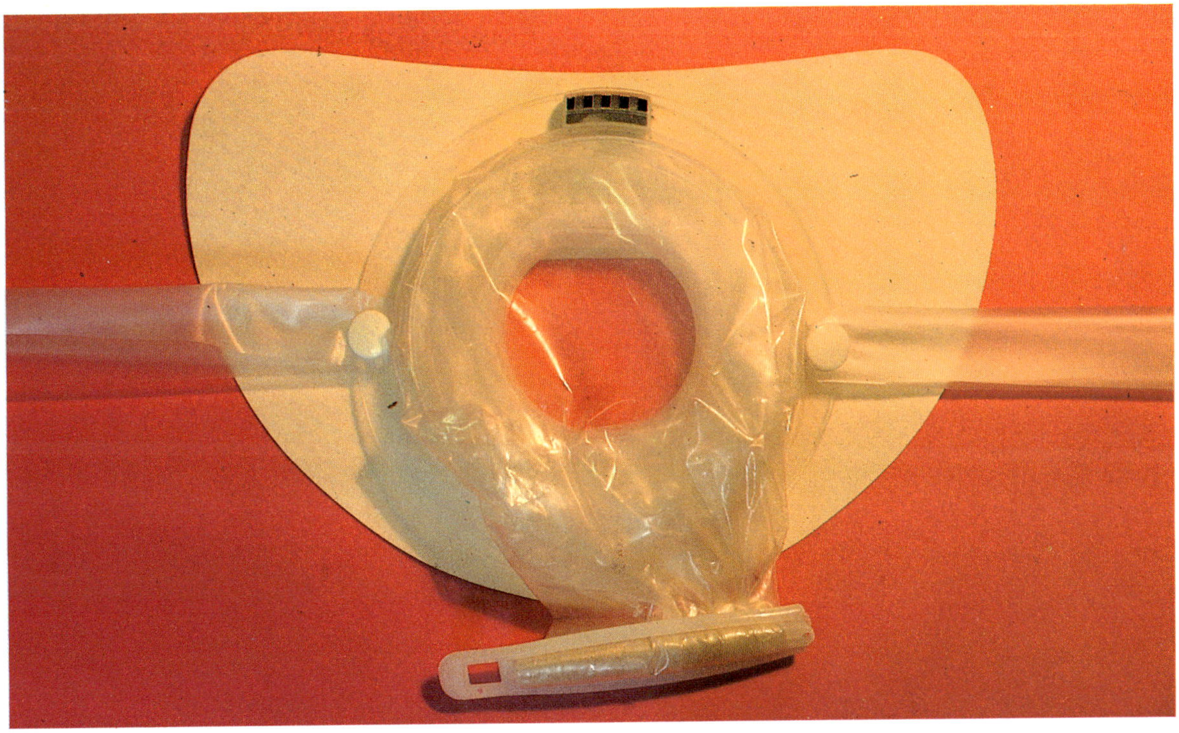

217 The complete appliance showing the cylindrical seamless pouch pleated over a low-profile spool mounted on a shield-like plate. The special clip holds the open end of the pouch firmly. Note the air filter at the top of the appliance.

218

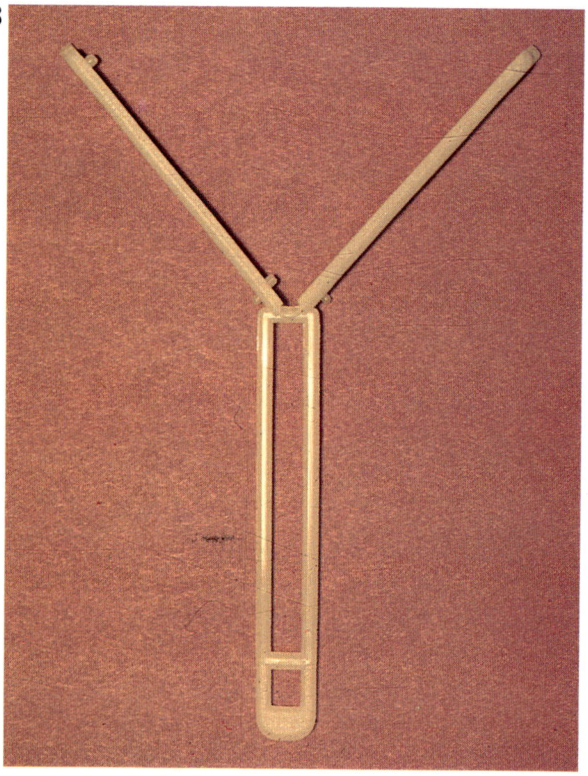

218 The open end of the pouch is carefully wound around the studded limb of the V-formation, after which the two limbs are impacted. The complex so formed is then pressed into the frame provided. This results in a very secure unit.

219

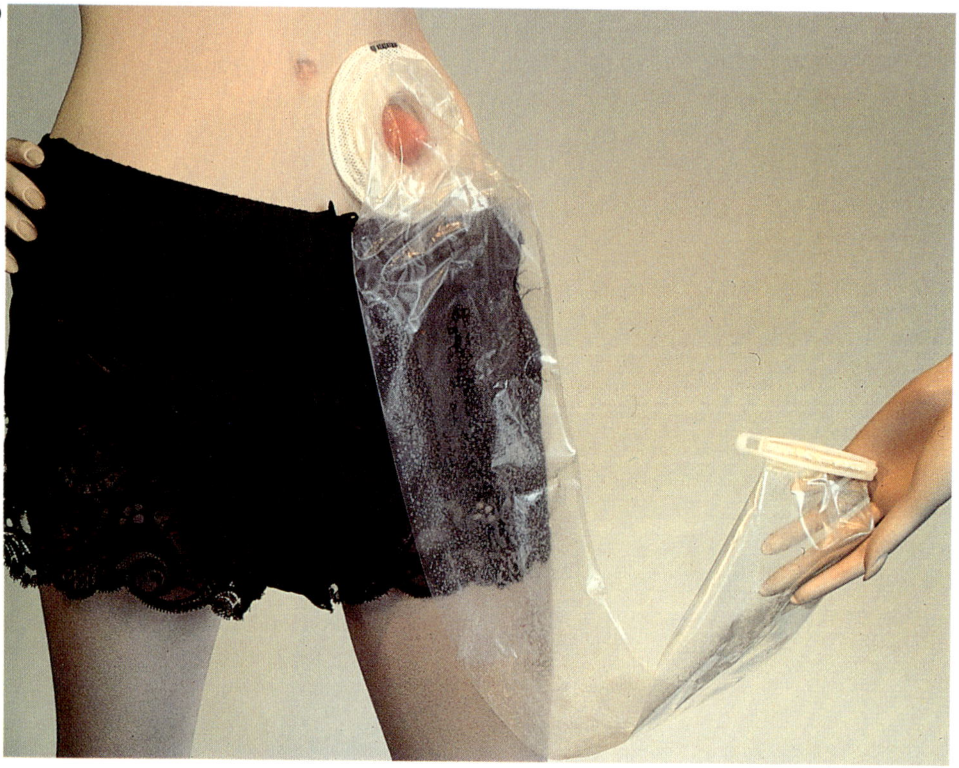

219 The fully drawn out pouch showing its usable length of over two feet. It is made of a thin sheet of plastic material, which has a high tensile strength.

Useful Addresses

Associations Etc.

Colostomy Welfare Group	38/39 Eccleston Square London SW1V 1PB
Ileostomy Association of Great Britain and Ireland	Amblehurst House, Cobham, Woking, Surrey GU24 9PZ
International Ostomy Association	Mr C.W. Beadle, General Secretary I.O.A., 5, 100 West State Road, Middle Ville MI 49333, U.S.A.
World Council of Entero-stomal Therapists	Assistant Director of Nurses /E.T., Princess Margaret Hospital for Children P.O. Box D.184 G.P.O., Perth, Australia.

Appliance Suppliers

		Code Letter
Coloplast International A/S	Bronzevej 4, DK 3460 Espergaerde, Denmark	C
Eschmann	Peter Road, Lancing, W. Sussex BN15 8TJ	E
Hollister Inc.	2000 Hollister Drive, Libertyville, IL 60048 U.S.A.	H
	Distributors outside Canada and U.S.A.: Abbott International Ltd., Abbott Park, North Chicago, Illinois 60064, U.S.A.	
Salt & Son Ltd.	220 Corporation Street, Birmingham B4 6QR	Sa
Simpla Plastics Ltd.	Phoenix Estate, Caerphilly Road, Cardiff CF4 4XG	Si
E.R. Squibb & Sons Inc. (Worldwide Headquarters)	P.O. Box 4000, Princeton NJ 08540, U.S.A.	Sq

Index

Abdominal incisions 64
– subcuticular stitch 64
– use of buttons 64, 65
Adhesives/removers 128
Allergy – *see* contact dermatitis
Amussat, Zuléma 8,10
Amylase 12
Antibiotics – *see* drugs
Anti-depressants – *see* drugs
Appliances –
– choice 45, 46, 47, 48
– early types 116, 117
– Koenig-Rutzen 120
– modern types 119–127
– protective rings 123
– St. Mark's cups 118
– skin protectives 127
– trusses 118

Belts 121, 126
Biethium 53
Bleeding 88, 89
Blockers – *see* drugs
Brooke, Bryan 9, 38

Cabbage 132
Caecostomy 14, 70
Codeine Phosphate – *see* drugs
Colitis – *see* ulcerative; Crohn's
Colonic polyposis 18, 19, 20, 21
Colostomy –
– double-barrel 52, 53
– indications 16
– magnetic 68, 134
– transverse 13, 49, 50, 51
Colostomy support rods 132
Colostomy Welfare Association 137
Contact dermatitis 100, 104, 105, 107
Continent ileostomy – *see* Kock's
Corticosteroids 105, 106, 134
Crohn's disease 27 –
– anal involvement 27
– fistula 27, 60, 62
– histology 28
– radiology 28
Cucumber 131

Detachment 90, 91, 92
Deodorants 129
Dermatitis –
– insult 99, 101, 102, 103
– contact 100, 104, 105, 107
– infective 100
Diet 131
Dilators, 118
Diphenoxylate – *see* drugs
Double-barrelled colostomy 52, 53
Drains 32, 33
Drugs, effects 129–131
Duret 8

Effluents 54
Eggs 131
Electrolytes 12

Familial polyposis – *see* polyposis coli
Fine 8
Fuestel 9
Fish 131
Fistula –
– anal 27, 60, 62
– stomal 93, 94, 95

Gangrene – *see* necrosis
Green vegetables 131

Hernia 108, 109, 110, 111, 112, 113
Herring 9
Hollister colostomy bags – *see* Appliances
Hollister irrigation set 129

Ileostomy –
– appliances – *see* Appliances
– continent 70, 71
– defunctioning 15
– effluent volume 12
– effluents 54
– reservoir 15
– siting 36
– temporary 15
– terminal 15
Ileostomy Association of Great Britain 137
Incisions 32, 33
Irrigation techniques 128

Kirschner 8
Kock 9
Kock's continent reservoir 70, 71
Koenig 9

Lavage 128
Laxatives – *see* drugs
Limòn, José 1
Littré 8
Lloyd-Davies 9
Lockhart Mummery 8
Luke, James 8, 114

Magnetic rings 68, 134
Mesenteric fixation 39
Miles 8
Muco-cutaneous sutures 42, 43, 51

Necrosis, stoma 78, 79, 80, 81
Nipple valve 70, 71

Omentum 61
Onions 131

Perineal wound –
– anal preservation 57
– closure 55, 56
– Crohn's 60
– dressing 56
– primary closure 55, 56
– semi-open 55, 58, 59
– types 55
– vagina 55, 58, 59
Pilloré 8
Polyposis coli –
– familial, macroscopy 18
– – microscopy 18
– – malignant change 19
– – radiology 19
– – stoma 66
– non-familial, histology 21
– – radiology 20, 21
Praxagoras 8
Prolapse 75, 85 87

Recto-colectomy 57, 62
Rectum –
– carcinoma 17
– histology 17
Retraction 82, 83, 84, 97
Rutzen 9

Sames 9
Schede 8
Stenosis 96, 97, 98
Steroid tape 105, 106, 134
Stoma –
– bleeding 88, 89
– caput medusae 66
– carcinoma in 69
– construction 34, 35
– hernia 108–113
– Kock's reservoir 67
– magnetic 68, 134
– necrosis 78–81
– prolapse 75, 85, 87
– retraction 82, 83, 84, 97
– site 29, 30, 31, 32, 74–77
– size 34, 36
– spout, fixation 39
– spout length 40, 41
– techniques –
– – muscle splitting 34, 35
– – trephine 36, 37
– suture material 133

Terminal colostomy, left iliac 13
Terminal ileostomy 12
Thiersch 8
Transverse colostomy 13
– construction 49, 50, 51
– double-barrel 52, 53
– defunctioning 14
– effluent 12, 49
– profile 12
– site 50
– split barrel 86
– use 49
Trephine opening 36, 37
Trypsin 12
Turnbull, Rupert 9, 72

Ulcerative colitis 22
– carcinoma 26
– crypt abscess 22
– histology 23
– radiology 23–25
– toxic megacolon 24

Vaginal excision 55, 58, 59
Vitamins B_{12} 12
– K 12

Water contents, of stoma 12